# FORTY YEARS

OF

# PSYCHIATRY

BY

WILLIAM A. WHITE, A.M., M.D., Sc.D.

**British Library Cataloguing-in-Publication Data**
A catalogue record for this book is available from the
British Library

# William Allen White

William Allen White was born on 10th February 1868, in Emporia, Kansas, U.S.A. He was a renowned American newspaper editor, politician, author, and leader of the 'Progressive movement' – a broad philosophy based on the idea of progress in human endeavours.

Soon after his birth, White's parents, Allen and Mary Ann Hatten White, moved to El Dorado, Kansas. He spent the majority of his childhood in this remote town, where he loved studying the animals and reading various books. White attended the nearby College of Emporia, and later, the University of Kansas. In 1892, after successfully graduating, he started work at *The Kansas City Star* as an editorial writer.

In his personal life, White married Sallie Lindsay in 1893. They had two children; William Lindsay, born in 1900, and Mary Katherine, born in 1904. It was also during the 1890s, that White developed a friendship with President Theodore Roosevelt, that lasted until the latter's death in 1919. They spent many nights visiting each other. Later, although White supported much of the New Deal (the president's series of domestic programs in response to the Great Depression), he voted against Roosevelt at every opportunity.

In 1895, White bought the *Emporia Gazette* for $3000 from William Yoast Morgan – and became its editor. He attracted national attention the following year, after a scathing attack on the Populists and William Jennings Bryan (an influential Democrat), titled 'What's the Matter with Kansas?' White sharply ridiculed Populist leaders for letting Kansas slip into economic stagnation and not keeping up economically with neighbouring states – because their anti-business policies frightened away economic capital. The Republicans sent out hundreds of thousands of copies of the editorial during the U.S. presidential election of 1896.

With his warm sense of humour, articulate editorial pen, and commonsense approach to life, White soon became known throughout the country. His *Gazette* editorials were widely reprinted, and he wrote syndicated stories on politics, as well as many books (White had twenty-two works published throughout his life). These included biographies of Woodrow Wilson (1924) and Calvin Coolidge (1925), and 'Mary White' – a touching tribute to his sixteen year old daughter on her death in 1921. He also wrote several fictional works, including *The Court of Boyville* (1899), *A Certain Rich Man* (1909), and *God's Puppers* (1916).

In his novels and short stories, White developed his idea of the small town as a metaphor for understanding social change and for preaching the necessity of community. While he expressed his views in terms of the small municipality, he tailored his rhetoric to the needs and values of emerging urban America. In his novel *In the Heart of a Fool* (1918), White fully developed the idea that reform remained the soundest ally of property rights. He felt that the Spanish-American War fostered political unity, and believed that a moral victory and an advance in civilization would be compensation for the devastation of World War One.

Based on ideas such as these, White became leader of the Progressive movement in Kansas, forming the Kansas Republican League in 1912, to oppose the railroads. In this role, he helped Theodore Roosevelt form the Progressive (Bull-Moose) Party in 1912 – in opposition to the conservative forces surrounding incumbent Republican president, William Howard Taft. White was also a reporter at the Versailles Conference in 1919, and a strong supporter of Woodrow Wilson's proposal for the League of Nations. The League went into operation but contrary to White's hopes, the U.S. never joined.

In 1924, angered by the emergence of the Ku Klux Klan in the state, he made an unsuccessful run for Kansas Governor. White was on the liberal wing of the Republican party, and wrote many editorials praising the New Deal of President Franklin D. Roosevelt. He was a key figure in supporting the presidential nominees, Alf Landon of Kansas in 1936, and Wendell Willkie in 1940.

The last quarter century of White's life was spent as an unofficial national spokesman for Middle America. This led President Franklin Roosevelt to ask White to help generate public support for the Allies, before America's entry into World War II. White was fundamental in the formation of the 'Committee to Defend America by Aiding the Allies', sometimes known as the 'White Committee'. He had to fight the powerful 'America First faction', which believed, like most other Republicans, that the U.S. should stay out of the war. White spent much of his last three years involved with this committee.

White visited six of the seven continents at least once in his long life. Due to his fame and success, he received ten honorary degrees from varying universities, including one from Harvard.

Sometimes referred to as the 'Sage of Emporia', he continued to write editorials for the Gazette until his death on 29th January 1944. White died in Emporia, Kansas – at the age of seventy-five. He has since been awarded many posthumous honours, and the town of Emporia honours him to this day with city limits signs on IH-35 announcing 'Home of William Allen White'. His autobiography, which was published posthumously, won a 1947 Pulitzer Prize.

# PREFACE

In presenting this book under the title "Forty Years of Psychiatry," my aim is to give a picture of my personal experience in this department of medicine. I shall not endeavor to present an exhaustive survey of the scientific field through this period with criticisms of the innumerable contributions which have been made from all parts of the world. This would be a stupendous task of perhaps dubious value. My aim is a much more personal and intimate one, from one point of view, and a much more general one, from another. I wish to show what has happened in these forty years as I have seen it, for during this time all the great developments in this field of medicine have taken place and I have seen them unfold before my eyes, and in many instances I have taken an active part in what has happened. It is not my aim, either, to present a book which is in any sense autobiographical. This again would be a task which, entirely for reasons other than its difficulty, I should hesitate to undertake. The object of my book will be one that lies somewhere between the two objectives suggested. I shall undertake to give in outline, and I trust in interesting narrative form, the main facts of the development of psychiatry as I have seen them during this period of forty years, and I shall preface this presentation only by such details about myself as are necessary to enable the reader to have some idea of the background and preparation and outstanding tastes of the person through whose eyes, as he reads these pages, he will view the drama of psychiatry.

Inasmuch as through the years I have never kept a record of events for the purpose of using them in this way, there will be perhaps instances in which the temporal sequences may be wrong or the definite dating inaccurate; but, as the reader may gather as he turns the pages, my real interest is not in such matters but in the functional development of the subject, and in this respect dates are often misleading as perhaps much further advance has taken place in one locality than in another. And so I beg the reader's indulgence if perchance his keen eyes detect such errors. Dates are after all most important oftentimes in merely fixing the attention upon some dramatic incident which shows the direction in which progress in certain respects is taking place. Almost invariably careful study of

such situations shows that there were many antecedents which prepared the way for this dramatic event, and that subsequently there
are many places in the world which have not been influenced by it.
This is true, for example, of the liberation of the "insane" by
Dr. Philippe Pinel in 1792 at the Bicêtre and following that in 1793
at the Salpêtrière, as set forth in the well known painting that hangs
in the latter institution. Pinel was by no means the first to treat the
mentally ill kindly or with understanding, and following his dramatic
liberation of them in this Parisian hospital many institutions could
be found in many parts of the world where they continued long after
to deal with their mental patients quite as cruelly and quite as
ignorantly as before. Nevertheless 1793 stands out in our minds
like a punctuation mark separating the age of ignorance and cruelty
from the age of humanitarian endeavor. In this respect the date is
important, but from the point of view of understanding the functional
significance of the tendency which it made visible it is by no means
of such outstanding significance.

W. A. W.

Washington, D. C.

# CONTENTS

# Contents

# CHAPTER I

## BACKGROUND AND TRENDS

I was born in the center of a large metropolitan area, the city of Brooklyn, in 1870, and my preliminary education was in the public schools of that city. Probably the facts of outstanding significance in those early years were, first, that the house in which I was born and lived was only half a block from a combined hospital and medical school, and from my earliest days I can remember the clang of the gong of the ambulance as it stood in front of the gates demanding admission for some poor injured soul who was being brought to the hospital. I can also remember how, from time to time, the blood-soaked straw mattresses were stacked up in the yard of this hospital and burned, and how we youngsters used to gather around the gate and watch the bonfire and probably experience all sorts of vague and ill-defined emotions. Among my principal playmates of that day were the sons of the Professor of Surgery, so that in a somewhat surreptitious way I was enabled to gain access to the grounds of the hospital and to see a good deal that was going on there. I presume I made myself somewhat of a nuisance about the accident rooms and the dispensary, and I occasionally ventured to the top floor in the college part and inspected the dissecting room and its gruesome inhabitants. Simultaneously with these experiences I was going to school and my intimate schoolmate and chum was a boy much older than I who had decided to study medicine at this very college, so that I absorbed undoubtedly a great deal of enthusiasm in this direction from him as well as from my other associations. When the grammar school was finished and I went to high school my principal interest soon manifested itself in the natural sciences, and I found myself picked out by the teacher to assist in preparing the lectures in physics and chemistry. With the study of physiology and my continued associations my determination to study medicine, which undoubtedly existed all this time, became definitely crystallized, and I had begun to think of this profession as a definite goal.

While I was still in the high school an opportunity came to take an examination for a scholarship at Cornell University. This would mean four years of free tuition, and as I was poor and probably could not have negotiated a university education had I had to pay the ordinary price of instruction, I eagerly sought the opportunity to take this examination, aided and abetted by my school-boy friend, who had relatives in Ithaca and knew the lay of the land there. The day of the examination came and I took it, and although I have always felt that I made a pretty miserable showing on paper, still, as the State of New York and the particular portion of it in which I lived was entitled to a certain number of scholarships and for some unknown reason the number of applicants was below that number, I squeezed through and obtained my scholarship. This happened, as I recall it, in the summertime when my parents were away in the country or had not yet returned, and it was my proud privilege to announce to them when they did get back that I was going to college. I was fifteen years old when the events happened as above recorded and I started all alone on the train for Ithaca and an education. I had great aspirations in this direction and some rather definitely formulated ideas. The association with the sons of the surgeon had been a very valuable one to me. The oldest son, particularly, was of a highly intellectualistic type; and I was stimulated through them and my other contacts and my fragmentary introduction to science in the schools to attempt to satisfy my own curiosity in these fields by reading. In some way, the history of which has escaped my memory, one of the most important things in my life, as I look back upon it, happened somewhere about this period. I was introduced to the works of Herbert Spencer. Here I apparently found precisely what I was looking for, an account of the universe from the points of view of the several sciences, and all put together into a coherent, well-knit philosophy of formulations consisting of general laws of universal application. Here was the key to unlock all knowledge, and I started off with this key in my possession, convinced that the secrets of Nature would be revealed to me. Perhaps the most significant single impression and the most invaluable one which I obtained from the reading of Spencer was that which I relate to his First Principles and which in my own words amounts to this: that there is a kernel of truth in everything no matter how false or absurd it may appear upon the surface, and that it is that kernel of truth which is of value; and therefore nothing is to be scorned because everything really possesses for the unprejudiced mind something invaluable, if one will take the trouble to try to find it.

My early days at the university were pretty difficult ones. I had burned my bridges behind me and I found myself pretty lonesome in a world about which I knew nothing and in which I felt very strange. The lowest age at which the university would admit students was sixteen. I was only fifteen. I could afford to take no chances because this was my great opportunity, so I bravely lied and registered myself as seventeen years of age. It can be seen, therefore, that I was considerably younger than the run of students; and as I came from a school system which, although it belonged to a great city, was entirely dislocated from any scheme of preparation for advancing its students to the next step in the university, I found myself loaded with conditions and taking subjects that were strange to me and which I could not understand. This particularly applied to language and mathematics. However, I struggled along, rooming for the first few months with my friend, who entered at the same time with me, and soon became immersed in the student activities. For the most part, I fear, they were mischievous activities.

During these years at the university I continued to head in the direction of medicine, stressing particularly in my studies the natural sciences, physiology, anatomy, chemistry, biology, geology, anthropology, with a sprinkling of language and literature, but more especially coming under the direct and immediate influence of inspiring teachers. From the first I found that I had to earn my living, or at least part of it, though my parents helped as generously as they were able to. So that I was occupied all day long, from early morning until the university closed in the late afternoon at five or six o'clock. One of the professors generously gave me work to do for which I received the munificent sum of fifteen cents an hour, which through the years was gradually increased, in accordance I presume with the importance of the work that I learned to do, to twenty and finally twenty-five cents. My chum, who continued to attend the university during these years, worked with me, he practically in the position of curator of the museum and I working in the same lines as his assistant. Such work as this, together with a little tutoring, went a considerable way toward paying my expenses.

The influences to which I was exposed were of course numerous and of different kinds but the inspiring features represented a continuity of influence in a fixed direction that never ceased. I am particularly thinking of the work with Professor Burt G. Wilder on the morphology of the brain, the work with Professor Simon Henry Gage in histology and embryology, the unfolding of the history of the earth's crust by Professor Henry S. Williams in his lectures on geology and paleontology, the inspiring teaching of Professor John

Henry Comstock in entomology, the fascinating work in the laboratories in botany and zoölogy, and last but not least the influence of Professor Jacob Gould Schurman, then head of the School of Philosophy, subsequently President of the University, and only recently retired from the Diplomatic Service as Ambassador to Germany. I can remember Schurman's first lecture on ethics, in which he stated that once upon a time in the old days an ideally educated man was a man who knew everything, because in those days it was possible for a single human mind to compass all that was known; but that now knowledge had increased to such an extent that this was far from possible, and therefore today the ideally educated man was the man who knew something of everything and everything of something. This, of course, fitted right into what I had gathered from reading Spencer, and from that moment I hung upon every word of this talented lecturer and teacher.

When I went to Cornell Andrew Dixon White was still President. I lived within a stone's throw of his house, and while I did not know him personally in those days I learned to know him in later years and to have the same sort of affectionate regard and worshipful adoration of him that most Cornell students have at some time in their careers. To me it was nothing short of marvelous to realize that I could sit and chat with a man who used to walk arm in arm with Bismarck when they were representing their respective countries in Saint Petersburg. It served to bring the past closer to me, to make me realize that characters that had been only historical names before had really been living beings that walked the earth like other men. I always had this feeling about these great historical characters, a feeling of vagueness almost as if they had never existed outside of the pages of history; and it was always difficult for me to realize that Napoleon died during my own father's lifetime, and that my father's father up to the time of his death had lived under every President of the United States from Washington to Arthur.

The Cornell University of those days was not so far removed from the days of the founder that his life and his doings were solely matters of history. His sons were students in the university while I was there, and several of the professors—Wilder, Comstock, and James Law in veterinary medicine—belonged to the original faculty that he had brought to that rather desolate spot to help him found a great university where " any man could find instruction in anything." Again you will see a sentiment appearing on all the university literature, which appealed to my Spencerian training, just as did Schurman's introductory lectures.

The years at Ithaca as they remain in my memory were pleasant and of inestimable value. I worked hard and I played hard, but I never could pass the examinations in mathematics nor in Latin and Greek and so I remained an optional student but I used up all my scholarship rights. At the end of the time, when nineteen years of age, in 1889, I entered the Long Island College Hospital Medical College, the one near which I was born, and with the help of the professor whose sons I had played with as a youngster I was again able to reduce the cost of instruction to the minimum and also to find a little work here and there, assisting at an operation, giving an anesthetic, reading to a doctor whose eyes had gone bad, all of which brought in something that helped along. I was in the last class that was permitted to graduate with only two years of instruction, although I took in addition a summer course between these two years. I was on the whole better prepared than the majority of my class and I went through these two years very creditably. I was fascinated by the work, but as I look back upon it I had to work very, very hard just as I had had to in college, from eight o'clock in the morning a lecture or a recitation or a clinic every hour until four or five at least in the afternoon and then back again at night for work in the dissecting room, so that my days began early and ended late, and even then I had to go home and study. So that when I graduated in 1891, just twenty-one years old, I was pretty thin and pretty pale.

My first job after graduation was that of ambulance surgeon at an emergency hospital and ambulance center which served the manufacturing and factory districts of the city. It was a pretty trying transition from the class-room to a job of this sort where my personal skill, capacity for judgment and quick action might mean life or death, and I felt this responsibility very keenly. In fact I can remember that when I took the job over, for some reason which can only be explained by the perversities of fate, there was a period of something like two or three days when no ambulance call came in at all—a length of time unheard of before without a call being received. During this time I spent my hours wondering what I would do and if I could do it at all and really becoming progressively more scared of what the first call held for me, but in due course this passed and I learned that even the life of an ambulance surgeon, who presumably deals only with emergencies, can for the most part sink into a rather deadly routine, and before I was through with it we young doctors would be sitting around Saturday night matching small coins or making miniature bets as to what the next case would be, in order apparently to add a little excitement to an otherwise dull routine.

However, it is interesting, to me at least, that the things that stand out in my mind as a result of this experience are a few events of outstanding dramatic power and coloring. There was the call to the wharf, where a tramp steamer had just finished unloading and her steel hulk rose high above the wooden pier. Climbing into this old ship, I found the bodies of three men who evidently had been standing on one of the hatches, which had not been properly fixed and which had tilted with them and dropped them 'way, 'way down into the steel hulk of the ship, smashing them to bits. One of them was still alive. We strapped him to a couple of planks nailed together, hoisting his body with the donkey engine over the side of the ship on to the wharf. There was the priest with his vestments all on waiting for him, with a crowd of onlookers standing about with heads bared while the last sacraments of the church were administered to this poor wretch, and against the background of the whole the ambulance and the white horse, as I stood on the deck and watched— a picture never to be forgotten, containing the concentrated significance of life and of death and of religion, all expressed in the space of a few moments. And then there were those fine men who went down in a gas tank to make a repair, and somebody must have lighted a match or struck a spark, for the oil ignited, blew away their means of exit and left them in there in a mass of flames. When we got them out they were burned in parts of their bodies to a crisp, and one poor fellow begged me as hard as he knew how to kill him and put him out of his agony. I learned then that even morphine was not supreme against pain. Only one of them did I take to our hospital—a great big giant of a fellow who did not want to die and fought with all the strength he had for a week or more, swathed from head to foot with bandages that we unwound to apply fresh dressings every few hours. He had a sweetheart who used to come to see him and for whom he wanted to live, but the inexorable result of the surface burning of a large portion of the body, including breast and abdomen and face and arms, could not be indefinitely forestalled and he had to lose the fight. There was the little boy I found in a drugstore one afternoon sitting bolt upright in a chair, white as a ghost, with great big wide eyes. As I stepped in I wondered what was the matter with him, and then I looked on the white marble of the floor beneath and saw a little pool of blood. I learned that he had been run over by a street car, and when I picked him up in my arms to take him to the ambulance one leg dangled by a mere shred of flesh. The thigh had been cut through high up and the pelvis crashed into by the wheel of the car. I lay beside him in the ambulance watching for fear one of the big vessels might break loose; but it did not and we got him in bed. We sent for his mother and watched him gradually slip away. There is no end to these stories. I tell them to remind the reader and myself of what seems to be a fact. From the very first this interest in the drama of life was really an interest in life itself and in living beings, a type of interest which has been with me from the beginning and still is.

This ambulance work on alternate months, and in between work as house surgeon attending to the accidents as they were brought to the hospital or drifted in from one source or another, I finally felt had given me all it could and my next step, after about six months here, was to take an appointment on Blackwell's Island. Here I was to see life from another angle. I was on the Alms and Workhouse staff. I live in the old almshouse hospital, went to sleep every night to the strains of a German band playing in a beer garden just across the river, and took my meals in the workhouse where we were waited upon by a convict. We were rowed back and forth over the river by a group of prisoners in charge of a keeper. At one end of the island was the penitentiary, at the other end was the insane asylum, and we were in between. The organization of these New York islands has changed very much but I have no doubt they are still, as they were then, the repositories of the failures and the disappointments of one of the greatest cities of the world, who finally landed there to spend their last days and to die and be buried in Potter's Field. It was a gruesome business, this life with these poor people, who had long since given up hope, who were devoid of any of the ambitions or normal curiosities or intelligent interests of the rest of the world, who just sat there and sat there and sat there, eating their miserable food and waiting for death. And when death came in one of the old poorhouse wards, if it was in the night the priest was sent for, he administered the rites of the church, he closed the eyes, folded the arms on the breast and placed a Testament thereon, and the old women in the beds on either side went on sleeping. And in the morning two idiots—one known as Nosey because of his large nose, and the other as Johnny the Horse because of his playful way of dangling a bit of rope behind him as a tail and galloping about like a horse—came and put the body in a coffin-like receptacle and carried it off to the mortuary amidst the cynical comments of the other members of the ward made to one another to the effect that " It will be your turn next," etc. The dead-house was piled high with coffins, empty and full. Every day we went there to do autopsies, and the old fellow who had charge of it slept there on a bench right along with all this discarded human material. To cap it all, whenever a new and uninitiated doctor came on the staff and sent alcohol to the dead-house to preserve some of the organs that were removed at autopsy this old fellow would drink it; and one of my first experiences was to be waked up in the small hours of the morning by this same old chap with a "touch of the horrors," trembling and sweating and wanting help.

This life on the Island did not offer much except its drama, but there was plenty of that. I remember the grim humor of a fellow who would come to me and say he needed some medicine for this or that, adding, "For God's sake, Doctor, don't give me anything to give me an appetite"; and the tall, gaunt, thin, grotesque Don Quixote type of fellow who paraded up and down the grounds with a short, fat Sancho Panza type—such queer allegiances as this might have stepped out of the pages of Gustave Doré's illustrations. I went about the wards of the poorhouse every morning, like as not seeing when I first arose a stream of stretchers that had been brought down by a little steamer that made its rounds from island to island and from the city. These stretchers contained the patients that were sent over from the hospitals in the city, most of them fatally ill and some dying, sent to us to make room for other patients and, I always suspected, to reduce the death rate in the respective hospitals. Nothing was more pathetic than to see some poor chap taken out of his death-bed and transferred to the Island. There was no history with him, nothing—he was just a nameless, dying man about whom we knew only that which we could find out, we, an inexperienced lot of students just out of college. Then later on in the day there were the rounds of the dark cells of the workhouse, where prisoners had been put for discipline, in absolute darkness, with bread and water, a blanket and a bucket. Here were life and death reduced to their simplest, in the raw as it were. There was no visiting staff except on paper, no intelligent direction, the whole great piece of municipal machinery apparently conducted solely on the principle of economy.

There was not much here for me to learn. I stayed only a short time and then accepted a vacancy on the medical staff at the old college hospital where I had graduated and where I would be closely supervised, directed and instructed by a competent force of interested teaching, visiting physicians. I finally sought out by this circuitous route the sort of thing that I needed, and the months spent here were spent to great advantage. Life and death here too were both very close. The obstetrical wards and the dead-house were not far apart. The hospital was an old one like hundreds of hospitals throughout the country in those years and the nursing force was competent, but it had responded to a demand which after all was of only a few years' growth. Antiseptic surgery was carried out in all its details in one part of the institution, and in another the operation was performed on the same table that the professor of anatomy used for demonstrating his dissections. There were all sorts of differences of degree of cleanliness and differences of technique of one sort or another, but the staff were all interested, were all earnest, were all teachers and were inspiring, and these months were very helpful. I shortly associated myself particularly with a dispensary service that had to do with nervous diseases and made a friend of Dr. William Browning, who conducted that room and who remains one of the outstanding neurologists of the country. Then the day came when Dr. Browning was asked by his friend, Dr. G. Alder Blumer, Superintendent of the Utica State Hospital, if he knew a young man who would be suitable for him to appoint. Dr. Browning recommended me. I drew all the money I had in the world out of the bank and went to Albany to take the Civil Service examination. I was No. 4 on the list so Dr. Blumer could not appoint me, but his previous first assistant, Dr. Charles G. Wagner, had just gone to Binghamton and Dr. Blumer recommended me to him; and I was soon faring forth again alone on a railroad train, wondering what lay at the other end of the route.

# CHAPTER II

## My Introduction to Psychiatry

The railroad journey was not a long one, only some five or six hours, and when it ended it ended at the beginning of my contact with psychiatry.

I was prepared for the study of mental disease by my previous experience and was set in that direction. I had taken the first course ever given in physiological psychology at Cornell University, and I believe the second course of that character given in the United States. I had become interested in the brain through my studies of its morphology under Wilder and inspired by the teachings of Schurman in the department of philosophy and in psychology; and later on, in my internship, I had been particularly interested in the diseases of the nervous system as I saw them in the dispensary with Dr. Browning. To all of these experiences had been added my own particular bent of mind, conditioned to a considerable extent by my study of the Synthetic Philosophy of Spencer; and so when I arrived at the State Hospital at Binghamton I was prepared to take up the specialty of my choice.

I found myself in a new world that was very different from that which I had left, a hospital in name to be sure but with almost none of the characteristics of the hospitals with which I had been familiar. The buildings contained wards and the wards patients, but the patients for the most part were up and about and so far as I could see a large proportion of them had nothing in the world the matter with them. I remember my first walk through the wards with the Superintendent, Wagner, who introduced me to a patient. He asked the patient some questions and then turned to me and asked me whether I knew what was the matter with him. Of course I did not, and of course, also, the patient was a paretic and his speech disturbance was supposed to have been the obvious indication of that condition which I should have spotted. But in my medical student days I had had no instruction in psychiatry. We had had lectures and clinics in neurology, and Dr. John C. Shaw, who was the head of the department, had been the Superintendent of the large hospital for mental diseases at Flatbush, later taken over by the State; but the only patient that was presented during my two years where the question of the mental condition was raised at all was a patient presented by Dr. Shaw, who wound up in his discussion with the diagnosis that he was probably a malingerer.

When I went to Binghamton, therefore, I was ill prepared in this specialty in every respect except determination, enthusiasm and curiosity, and so I knew nothing about the patients in this new world. The hospital was beautifully located on a hill overlooking the Susquehanna Valley. Its main building, of stone, was one of the outstanding architectural successes of the State Architect's office. It was, as it seemed to me then, a tremendously big plant with many buildings and hundreds of acres of land and nearly a thousand patients. The previous Superintendent, Dr. Theodore S. Armstrong, had been a worthy representative of the times that were then passing. He had been picked for service because he was a successful country practitioner. He knew nothing much about mental illnesses but neither did anyone else. He was an honest, industrious representative of the interests of the state and of the patient, and he subscribed to the doctrines of kindness and non-restraint which represented the beginnings of the new period of humanitarian care which stretched away back to Pinel and which there is unfortunately still need of emphasizing in many quarters. Like most superintendents of his time, however, he was perhaps more interested in his farm, because he knew more about it, and this after all operated to the advantage of his patients because large numbers of them spent their days out of doors in the wholesome work of cultivating the soil. Armstrong, however, was dead, and a new Superintendent, Wagner, had come to take his place and had been there only a few months when I arrived. The new Superintendent was a young man of magnificent physique and great physical vigor, of enterprise and ambition and good medical and scientific training, and he was starting right off to change the old institution in accordance with his ideals. He had just done an amputation for gangrene, a thing probably unheard of in the old days before his arrival, and the patient not only survived but continued to live for many years afterward. I remember him very well, even his name. I doubt if he ever found out that his leg had been amputated.

In these early days when the Superintendent was busy remodeling here and rebuilding there, putting up new buildings somewhere else, arranging a dispensary service for patients who needed to have their eyes and ears and teeth fixed, keeping in mind the need for operating facilities and hydrotherapy, I was busy getting oriented. The library of the hospital was small but I went through it pretty systematically and it was not infrequent that the dawn found me in the office poring over such books as were at my disposal. There are perhaps two lasting impressions about that period. One was that about the only virtue that I was able to discover in the state hospital as an agency for the application of therapeutics to the mentally ill was that the patient who came there had been removed from the conditions under which his psychosis developed. This I felt to be a very important feature in what might be called the treatment, and a very significant factor in recovery. I still think it is, though I never see anyone mentioned it. Another thing I learned was that if I really wanted to know something about a patient I did not ask the doctor. I asked the supervisor, the man who had been in charge of some half dozen wards for the preceding twenty years, and who had had daily, frequent, personal contacts with the patient ever since his admission or for a long period of years. The intelligent supervisor knew a lot of things about the patient. He could tell what he would do under a given set of circumstances, how far he could be trusted, whether he was telling the truth or not, and a hundred other things that the physician did not know even though the physician gave his discussion of the patient the color of a scientific discourse. The young men and women who came to us from the surrounding countryside to care for these patients were on the whole a fine lot, and although they had not been trained in nursing care, nor anything else for that matter, they had that most important of all characteristics, that fundamental essential for dealing with sick people, particularly the helplessly sick—they had character.

As I have said, there were no nurses, there were no ward employees who had any systematic training whatever in these first years, and the care of the patients, while it was intended to be kindly and while abuse was never tolerated for a moment, was in its practical results very far from what we would consider today adequate care. Where we failed in those days most completely was, of course, where we are apt to fail most today; namely, in the care of the violent and dangerous patients, on the one hand, and of the feeble, demented and bedridden, on the other. Mechanical restraint was for the most part taboo although we did use from time to time the restraining sheet—a perfectly hellish contrivance, literally speaking, in hot weather; and I am sure I have seen at least one patient die from heat exhaustion as a result of it. Chemical restraint, however, was freely resorted to, and under the care of one of the physicians in particular the patients were regularly doped with a mixture of chloral and bromide that kept them in a semi-stuporous condition, which I am sure has everything to be said against it and nothing to be said for it. I remember very well during my residence on Blackwell's Island how in the small hours of the morning when I came back from the city in the row-boat and landed at the pier at the asylum end of the Island, I could look back a distance of a few hundred feet and see the building where the women patients were confined. My memory of that vision is a building in which each window was a glare of light, and I can hear now the sounds that issued therefrom which reminded me of a hive of bees. These disturbed women, as they were called, were obviously in a state of continuous noisy activity all night long, and yet they were the patients who received bromide, chloral and some derivative of hyoscyamin regularly throughout the twenty-four hours. Their condition, I suspect—I never was in that building that I can recall—was probably one of semi-delirium. Today, with the practical abolition of the use of such drugs, the grounds of the mental hospital are as quiet at night as any country suburb.

The other group of patients where good intentions had to replace knowing how in their care were the patients in the infirmary wards. I can still see these very terrible places in which in a single ward forty or fifty bed-fast patients were cared for. These were the days before the connection between syphilis and general paresis had been disclosed, and many of these patients were terminal paretics. Others, of course, were seniles, hemiplegics, with a fair sprinkling of low-grade idiots. These bed-fast patients if they were old and feeble pretty generally developed bed sores; and the paretics characteristically developed them, so that it was not unusual to see a paretic die emaciated to a mere skeleton, with bed sores from the back of his head to his heels exuding literally pints of pus a day. This sort of thing fortunately has become past history in well administered institutions, and I have not personally seen a bed sore for years, but we presumed in those days that this sort of exitus was inevitable and that the bed sores were due to disturbances in the functions of the trophic nerves. We had similar mystical explanations for cauliflower ear, which used to make its appearance from time to time, particularly on our wards where we had disturbed patients. I can say also that I have not seen a cauliflower ear for years except it belonged to a boxer or wrestler who happened to be admitted to the hospital with one.

These big wards filled with these helpless, bedridden people, senile, deteriorated, or " demented " as we then said, to the point of living practically only a vegetative existence, filthy in their habits, and exuding pus in many instances from extensive denudations over the bony surfaces of the back, presented a picture of filth and degradation and human suffering that can hardly be imagined. If any of these patients refused food they had to be tube-fed twice a day; and during the broiling heat of midsummer these wards were infested with flies and one can imagine under these circumstances that they must have been terrible places to work in. The wonder was that we could get faithful employees to take care of this class of patients in these surroundings, working as they did twelve and fourteen hours a day. One of the outcomes of these conditions was undoubtedly the fact that patient after patient died in these surroundings with a hemorrhagic form of dysentery, and as I did all the autopsies at one time I learned to expect this condition, to find the mucous membranes almost black with contained blood. The dead-house offered the easiest and most natural entrée to scientific interest in our patients. We had not yet learned anything worth while of their psychology.

Early in our new Superintendent's career, however, a training school for nurses was established which had as its objective the teaching of the rudiments of nursing to those who had the immediate care of the patients. I believe I gave the first course of lectures in that school, and I continued to teach for a number of years. It will be recalled that I had previously helped prepare the lectures for the professors in the high school, that I had done the same sort of thing plus tutoring at the university, and I had also taught in the medical college, having been picked out of the class to help demonstrate in obstetrics on the mannikin. So I enjoyed this teaching experience, and of course the result was to improve the standard of care of the patients, particularly on the wards where they were helpless and physically ill. There were no specially provided wards for physically ill patients except the infirmary wards that I have just described. Here nursing care was needed as it was also in the reception wards, to which patients who were physically ill were not infrequently admitted. Elsewhere in the institution patients who became physically sick were cared for wherever they happened to be, for the most part, and cared for by the physician in charge of the service. There was no operating room, for example, and when an operation had to be performed, and it was very rare that necessity pushed us to this extreme, a room had to be dismantled and completely prepared for this purpose and a visiting surgeon brought in to operate. Occasionally a gangrenous limb or an acute appendix would force this issue. Otherwise, however, patients lived or died with what ailed them with very little assistance from surgery.

It will be seen from the descriptions thus far that a typical and well conducted hospital for mental disease of this period had really very little idea, according to our present standards, of what it was all about. The Superintendent in this case, as in the other cases of which I knew, was a kindly man who was fully convinced of the wisdom of the humanitarian doctrines and committed to carrying them out to the extent that he was able to intelligently translate them into action. Here of course was the weak point, for what to do with a violent patient except to restrain him physically or chemically no one knew. And how to improve the conditions of the infirmary ward was in general another mystery so long as we were dominated by theories of trophic nerves and the like. Kindness, however, was the keynote, and the energy which is expended in a modern hospital in many diverse activities was then concentrated largely on good housekeeping and the wards were spic and span in every respect. Unfortunately, of course, conditions in other institutions and localities here and there in the United States nowhere approximated these, and the tales of neglect and cruelty, abuse and indifference, that came from those places made us realize that our efforts in the humanitarian direction were still needed.

About the time of my appointment on the State Hospital staff the State of New York passed its State Care Act. This act provided that the insane should be taken care of by the State, which meant that they were to be taken out of county houses in particular, to say nothing of jails; and in pursuance of this act each state hospital had designated a certain number of counties immediately surrounding it, which comprised its district and from which it took the "insane." It was the very excellent practice in those days to send a nurse for the patient. Previously the patients had been transferred to the hospital by the county authorities or someone else, and it was not an infrequent experience to have them brought tied up in all sorts of ways, chained even, and handcuffed. We were able to develop nurses in this work so that the transfer of the patient to the hospital in a kindly, comfortable manner and with promises of help was assured. From time to time when the nurses were on these trips they found the patient particularly unruly or very ill; or the commitment papers, which were sent ahead of the patients before the hospital sent for them, disclosed certain conditions which made it desirable to send a physician on these trips. I have covered pretty well the central and southern part of New York State, and in doing so I came in contact in the early days with the remnants of the old county care system. It was a deplorable system, indeed, in which the ruling idea was economy. Poormasters boasted of how little they could support their inmates upon, and the medical attention was confined to the occasional visit of a nearby country doctor, which meant of course in the long run that the patients were systematically neglected and that ignorance ruled the entire system. The State Care Act was a most benevolent move in the direction of better care. It recognized the fundamental principle that the county or the municipality, as the case might be, was too small a political subdivision to undertake the problem of the care of the " insane." The economic burden was too great and it was essential that the state should take it over in order to insure adequate care. This the state did and it resulted in the development of the great state hospital system, which, of course, in the early days was pretty cruelly criticized in some instances by outsiders as being nothing but a great hotel system for boarding the patients. It was not appreciated that the environment of the hospital, quite unconsciously probably but nevertheless actually, developed along simpler lines in which individuals of inadequate make-up could live much more peacefully and function much more effectively: that the whole movement in the direction of humanitarian care was a necessary precedent to the scientific era: that the administration of the hospitals, located as they were in country districts for the most part with adjoining large farms, provided after all the best sort of occupation that could be devised, particularly where the patients came largely from a farming community; and that these great institutions were really the foundations of the modern hospitals where scientific psychiatry is undertaken and practiced.

# CHAPTER III

## PROGRESS

Under the wise direction of the Superintendent the hospital took on more and more those qualities that one associates with an institution for the care of the sick. The training school developed and brought a more highly intelligent and better trained personnel to these duties; and the appointment of visiting physicians who spent half a day or so each week at the hospital enabled the patients to get care and treatment for disabilities due to diseases of the eye, ear, nose, throat and teeth. The remodeling of old buildings, the building of new buildings, the addition of facilities for medical care, the equipment of an operating room, the construction of an amusement hall— all of these things added to the ability of the institution to care properly for its sick patients, and to the interest and variety of the institutional environment which made for the contentment of the patients, and, what is at times almost equally important, of the relatives also.

During the first few years of my residence here the old ideas of mental illness, which had dominated so long, were still in existence, as they were elsewhere throughout the country. Patients were either maniacal or melancholic or demented. General paresis was occasionally diagnosed but there was no more than a suspicion, although at times a pretty strong one, that there was some connection between it and syphilis; and the mental examinations consisted of undirected conversations with the patient followed by brief notes written in ponderous case books by longhand. There was very little if any suggestion that the mental symptoms had any meaning back of them, that the psychosis was a reaction of the organism in any way, defensive, compensatory or otherwise. The whole situation was looked upon as being pretty much of a mystery, and there was hardly any light to be had on these questions from any source. Finally, however, the work of Professor Emil Kraepelin seeped through the barriers of ignorance and its results became known to us little by little. Like all new concepts, it resulted in a considerable awakening of interest not only in the patients but the old-time and oft-repeated efforts at classification received a new impetus. It must be remembered that in those days the requirements for appointment to the medical staff were not very high and had not very much to do with the particular problems presented by the care of the "insane." There was then, much more than now, a tendency to take a job in a state hospital just because it was a job and insured the incumbent a safe haven from the economic struggle for existence. Of course this same thing still maintains; but then there was no such thing as a practicing psychiatrist outside of an institution of this sort and no one ever thought of going to such an institution in order to fit himself to practice this medical specialty. The state hospitals were great, often walled, institutions that carried on quite apart from the general body of medical men, and the practitioners outside had little or no interest in the problems developed by the "insane." There was a pretty definite cleavage between the intra- and the extra-mural groups of physicians, with a tendency to accumulate in the state hospitals a certain considerable proportion of dead wood, physicians who routinely went through the motions but who had ceased to be progressive, in fact who did not know the lines along which progress lay. All this, of course, was naturally incident to a period in which there was no widespread information about mental disease, and even those who were on the firing line had not very much to offer. So that when the Kraepelinian ideas came along it was slow work finding their way through this barrier of indifference but when they did they produced a great quickening of interest.

During all this period my own interests seem to have been protected by some beneficent influence, for they never lagged and I continued my studies as energetically as ever. I also felt very definitely that the separation of the state hospital from the general medical fraternity, as I saw it, was very unfortunate, and I joined the local medical societies and kept as closely in touch with what they were doing as possible. I began also to write from time to time, more particularly to do abstract work. It was in these early days that I met my very dear friend, Dr. Smith Ely Jelliffe, of New York City, who was then, like myself, in the early years of the practice of his profession, and being somewhat short of funds incident to a growing family he attempted to kill two birds with one stone and combined his summer vacations with residence in interesting institutions. One summer brought him to Binghamton. He spent it at the State Hospital and we became then close friends and our friendship has continued until the present day. He was then an editor, and later on he acquired the *Journal of Nervous and Mental Disease* following the death of its then owner and I became one of its constant contributors. He sent to me exchange journals from foreign countries which I abstracted regularly each month—a tedious and at times a somewhat grilling task but one which I kept up conscientiously for years, and I found that it repaid the effort that I put into it. In fact in those days the literature of mental disease was exceedingly scanty even in the foreign journals, and the number of books available to us in this country in English was very small. The first book that I read, I remember, was Savage, and then later we had Spitzka and Clouston and Bevan Lewis, and then the translation of Kirchhoff, followed, of course, in ever-increasing number by works from the pens of psychiatrists in various parts of the world. But to begin with it was all very meager and the work on the foreign journals was very helpful.

In the late '90's a number of very important and significant things happened. In the first place, the whole trend of hospital care had been very materially changed in its immediate objectives. The state hospital instead of being merely a large hostelry had undertaken to try in fact to be an actual hospital; and in New York State, largely under the leadership of Dr. Peter M. Wise, Superintendent at Ogdensburg, followed by Dr. William Mabon, there was a definite effort to treat the patients quite as they would be treated in a general hospital. They were received and put to bed and regularly examined by routine methods, just as if they were there for some physical illness. They were cared for by nurses who had been trained in the hospital training school; and the physicians who went about the wards instead of perfunctorily doling out sedatives or cathartics were now seen with thermometers in their vest pockets and with stethoscopes hanging about their necks. The theory, perhaps not very well formulated and not altogether conscious, was that in some way mental illness was related to physical disorder, and that if the physical disorder could be discovered and corrected the mental illness would take care of itself. This transition period in which the state hospital undertook, as it were, to imitate the general hospital was productive of a great deal of good because it fixed the training school as a permanent training institution; and it also insured the discovery of physical disease when it actually existed, and tended in the direction of instituting proper general medical practices for its correction. So that as a result of this movement general medicine gained a much firmer foothold in the hospital for mental disease. Unfortunately, however, no miracles happened as a result, and the patients did not get well in large numbers in consequence of this treatment. But the hospitals did become more orderly and better disciplined medical institutions and the patient was projected more definitely into the focus of attention of the management and particularly of the doctor. Much more was learned about him, not only physically but incidentally mentally, because it was impossible to have this closer contact without learning something all along the line.

When Dr. Wise left the Superintendency of the Ogdensburg State Hospital and Dr. Mabon took his place, Wise became the Commissioner in Lunacy of the State of New York and carried forward his ideas in that position in a way to involve the entire state hospital system. There was created by the Commission the Pathological Institute of the New York State hospital system, which was housed in New York City in the then recently completed Metropolitan Building on Madison Avenue. The Institute was located ten or a dozen floors up, had a magnificent suite of laboratories and offices and appointed a group of highly qualified men primarily engaged in research work, at the head of which was Dr. Ira Van Giesen, an enthusiastic and well equipped research worker with a keen, alert and interested mind that grasped in a comprehensive way the wide ramifications in the collateral sciences of the psychiatry of that day. Very shortly Wise was replaced by Dr. Frederick Peterson (1901), who brought to his Commissionership the mind of a highly trained neuropsychiatrist. During his Chairmanship the Institute came under the able administration of that most notable of American psychiatrists, Dr. Adolf Meyer, and became a place not only for research work but was also used as a sort of clearing-house for information for the various state hospitals, to which queries or pathological material might be sent and from which information and assistance might be expected. It also acted as an educational center to which members of the staffs of the various New York State Hospitals were sent from time to time for special study.

My own connection with the Institute was for me a very significant one. Dr. Boris Sidis had been picked out to head the Psychological Department and during a visit to New York City I went to the Institute to look it over and became acquainted with Dr. Sidis. A friendship immediately grew up between us and not long afterward I was using his methods and for the first time discovering that mental symptoms might have a meaning, that what the patient said and did had significance but that that significance could not be determined by the usual method of question and answer, that the real significance lay buried from the patient's vision as well as the doctor's and that special methods were required for determining it. The methods which we used in those days were the methods of hypnosis, or of what Dr. Sidis used to call the "hypnoidal state," which was closely allied. In these states of distraction we found our patients telling us all manner of experiences which they had passed through but which were shut off from their ordinary states of consciousness by an amnesia which made them inaccessible. Here, truly, was a fascinating field of study. I was entranced by what I found in my patients and I went back to the hospital filled with a determination to carry on experiments along these lines. I did this, and I spent a large portion of my time dealing with my patients according to this technique. It was an exceedingly interesting, valuable, and I believe crucial, experience for me personally. Almost without knowing it I absorbed the rudiments of what was subsequently to be the doctrine of the unconscious and accepted from the very beginning in my attitude toward these problems the principle of determination in the psychological field. The records of these earlier studies are in part contained in a book published in 1903 under the authorship of Dr. Sidis entitled " Psychopathological Researches in Mental Dissociation." Herein I have reported some of my experiences.

When I returned to the hospital with this point of view and started work there along the lines indicated I did not discover any very great enthusiasm on the part of my associates and none of them undertook any of the work of their own initiative. The state hospital physician in those days, as I have already indicated, was pretty apt to be a rather lazy sort of individual who got through the day with the least possible effort and looked forward to the time when he would have finished his rounds and could go downtown. While I was not by any means free from such inclinations, as I have already said some good spirit must have taken care of my fundamental interests and seen to it that they did not lag, because I very consistently kept at this work and turned out a number of publications bearing upon it.

The Pathological Institute continued to function for some time but its tendency was not actively in the direction of assisting the state hospitals or the members of the staffs thereof. Each member of the Institute tended to develop his own particular problems and interests and to be concentrated in their solution, so that later on a reorganization came to pass and new men stepped into the positions of control and the Institute was removed from its expensive quarters in the Metropolitan Building and took up its residence on Wards Island in one of the buildings belonging to the great hospital for mental diseases there, which had in the course of time been taken over by the state from the city. Here under the direction of Dr. Adolf Meyer, now Professor at Johns Hopkins, a more definite program of coöperation with the hospitals was worked out and the members of the staffs who showed particular interest were sent to the Institute for study. I had the privilege of being included in one of these groups and spent some time there with much profit. The Institute has continued to this day but is now very much elaborated as a part of the reception hospital situated in conjunction with the Medical Center in the City of New York.

I have outlined these various stages briefly, as above stated, with reference particularly to New York State, because, in the first place, I am much more familiar with what happened in that state, having been on the staff of one of its state hospitals, and, secondly, because what was happening there was indicative of the direction of progress, a direction which many of the states did not follow for a good many years but which nevertheless has in general been the direction which psychiatric progress has taken in this country. There was first the conscious adaptation of the humanitarian attitude: the doing away with restraint both physical and chemical: the turning of the asylum into the hospital and the making of this change a real one rather than a change in name only by carrying out the hospital regime and administering in accordance with hospital organization methods. Then following this an effort at introducing scientific research in all the various departments—anthropological, histopathological, chemical and psychological in particular, and in the latter field the uncovering of the tremendously significant fact that mental symptoms have meanings which can be disclosed by the application of properly worked out methods. All of this evolution took place naturally not only in a linear direction but in every direction, each new move necessitating a readjustment of the whole organization, the raising of the standards of the personnel throughout—not only the nursing personnel but the medical personnel, the introduction of medical and scientific interests seeping throughout the entire organization of the institution and tending to remold it all in a new form with objectives of care and treatment which accorded with the scientific principles that were found to be involved. Here really we see the inception of what was to be the development in psychiatry in the twentieth century.

# CHAPTER IV

## Transition from the Humanitarian to the Scientific

As I have already indicated and desire to impress still further upon the mind of the reader, the transition from one stage in the treatment of the mentally ill to the next took place very slowly and at different times in different places, and in some places these transitions have not yet occurred. So the change from the old, cruel days when the "insane" were treated on the theory that they were possessed of devils and the like and even in later days when they were treated in institutions by the devices that are described in the historical record of those times such as surprise baths of cold water, turning chairs, restraint in various kinds of cages, chairs, straitjackets, camisoles, and all such methods, to the humanitarian days of Pinel and following was one that was spread over many, many years and unfortunately has by no means been completed even now.

The transition from the humanitarian to the scientific period, which I dwelt upon somewhat in the last chapter, was also an exceedingly slow process that took place at different times in different places but was on the whole characterized by the same phenomena wherever it occurred. Perhaps in this country the outstanding original move in this direction was the effort of the Superintendent at the Utica State Hospital, Dr. John P. Gray. He was apparently convinced that the secret of mental disease would be found in the brain, and he got a brain pathologist and set him up in business at the hospital. Here interminable sections of the brain were made and were stained, hoping against hope that the secret would be discovered, that the physical basis of the patient's symptoms would disclose itself in a visible pathology of brain structure, particularly cortical structure. This period has been facetiously referred to as the period of "brain mythology." Those who were engaged in it never thought of questioning their basic premises and were convinced that if they failed to find what they were looking for it was only because their methods were not sufficiently refined, an excuse that we still hear. It is the favorite alibi today, as it was then, although now we hear it more frequently from the mouths of the chemists.

Of course in those days the methods of the histological examination of brain tissues were exceedingly crude as compared with those of today, and the structure of the nervous system as disclosed by the microscope was hardly more complex than that which we find now in an ordinary textbook on psychology, the writer of which feels impelled, for some mysterious reason, to present some chapters upon the structure of the nervous system. But for the most part it was as true then as it still is that people find what they are looking for and not what they are not looking for, and so it was necessary to go through a long period of evolution in order that the questions that the histopathologist asked of the tissues that he was examining under the microscope might undergo very considerable changes and as a result he might find very different things from those found by his predecessors. At any rate this method of investigation dominated the field, so far as there was a field, for many years, and the state hospitals at the beginning of the present century felt that they were living up to what was expected of them if they incorporated a laboratory along with the dead house, in which the tissues of the patients autopsied could be examined microscopically, particularly the nervous tissues. A dead house pathology was the opening wedge for the entrance of science into the study of mental disease, as it had for a long time been a standby in general medicine. It was natural that with the effort to solve the problems presented by the mental patient in a scientific way the methods of the general hospital should be imitated. When the cruel methods of the past were displaced by the sympathetic attitude of the humanitarian period the fundamental assumption was that the " insane " person was a sick person. Therefore, if he was sick he must be treated in a hospital, and the only hospitals that had arrived at a significant development were those for bodily diseases and it was but natural that they should be copied, despite the fact that during this period body and mind were still thought of as in two separate categories. There seemed to be no other direction in which to go. And so just as the scientific effort took on the color and proportions of the efforts that had been made in general medicine and established a dead house pathology with the hope that something might be discovered that was worth while, so the changes outlined in the last chapter in the care of the patient took on the characteristics of the efforts that were made in general hospitals to treat the physically ill. It is easy enough to feel out of conceit with these efforts, to look upon them as naïve or unscientific, or to call them by any disagreeable name that one may choose to think up; but it is difficult to see, as one looks back over the situation, just how the development could have been expected to take any other course. It was the natural evolution of the ways in which people thought about the mentally ill, and, as I have always contended, the way in which we think about things is the most important factor in scientific advance. It is the only direction, after all, in which we can look for broadened horizons, new orientations, different ways of asking questions of Nature. And so in correspondence with these concepts the asylums became hospitals, the hospitals acted as if they were treating bodily diseases and undertook their research problems from the point of view of autopsy material. The gain by these methods, despite the fact that they were valuable academically only as transitions, was very great in many directions, as already indicated. These gains can best be expressed by saying that all along the line a more intelligent personnel was brought into the situation, and that of course the result of a more intelligent personnel interested from various points of view, scientific as well as humanitarian, resulted in a more active interest in the individual patient and the individual patient naturally benefited as a result. He benefited principally by an improvement in his environment, not only an improvement in his personal environment because his nurses and doctors were better qualified but also an improvement in his physical environment because with this new interest there began to be an active effort to do something for the patient, and developments along the two broad lines of amusement and occupation were the result.

When it is remembered that about the same time that these changes were occurring physiological psychology was becoming a fact and the work of Kraepelin was becoming known, we can see that as in all movements of like significance changes were being effected in collateral regions of thought which bore more or less, directly or indirectly, upon the problems in hand. Psychology was breaking loose from its attachments to philosophy and metaphysics and under the control of the Wundtian school was rapidly becoming an experimental science, while Kraepelin was working at the psychology of his patients from the point of view of their symptomatology, and studying their diseases with an attitude closely resembling that of the biologist, namely, he was studying his patients' diseases not in cross-section, as had been the rule up to his time, but in longitudinal section, and his method according to his own description was the method of the study of the course of the disease and its outcome. By such a method he obtained results that were similar to those of the biologist in this respect: just as no biologist in the early days of Aristotle, for example, would have suspected butterflies and caterpillars to have any relation to each other, nevertheless if one studies their life history this relationship becomes apparent, so by studying the life history of the psychoses conditions that had previously been supposed to be entirely unrelated to one another were found to be just as organically a part of the total picture as the butterfly and the caterpillar. This result came about more especially in Kraepelin's delimitation of the manic-depressive psychosis. Previously the depressions and the excitements had been considered as separate entities, but it became obvious from Kraepelin's studies that they belonged together under the same classification. The psychology of the patient, which came to be called "abnormal psychology" and later on "psychopathology" began to develop in its own right, quite distinct from the academic psychology of the universities, which often, though it had become experimental, was, in its early stages at least, little more than a refined physiology of the special sense organs, and later was quite sterilized for the purposes of psychiatry because it hopelessly failed to take into consideration those aspects of the human being which are most significant—his hopes and his fears, his wishes and his frustrations, his ambitions and hatreds and loves, and all the rest of it—the things by which we know him and by which he endears himself to us or repels us. These were aspects of human nature which somehow seemed to have been forgotten, and the contact that I made with this aspect of the problem as I have already indicated in my association with Dr. Sidis was not taken up by others to any extent at all. In fact Morton Prince was almost the only man who took such matters seriously, with perhaps the exception of the psychologist, William James.

Here, then, was the state of affairs, roughly speaking, in the late '90's and the beginning of the present century. Definite scientific efforts were being made sporadically, here and there, but the humanitarian era was in the ascendant practically everywhere, at least lip worship was paid to its ideals even where those who were in command failed to have either the ingenuity, the intelligence, or the initiative to make these ideals come to pass in the actual conduct of their several institutions,—a very uneven and spotted development, but the sort of thing, it seems to me, that we always find, because after all development and progress is dependent, in its early stages at least, upon individuals and individuals can secure results only within the zones of their own influence. This was the transition period in this country, and abroad too, to the scientific study of the mentally ill and the translation of the results obtained from these studies into their care and treatment.

During these days I had continued to be fascinated by the problems presented by the patients. I practically lived on the wards among them, making rounds not merely in the morning and in the afternoon but pretty generally at night and often between times, so that I was on, at least the acute wards, not infrequently half a dozen times a day. I knew my patients individually and they all interested me, but I did not know how to ask them the questions that would throw light upon the problems they presented. I worked faithfully doing autopsies, staining tissues, making physical examinations, taking histories, and doing all the other things which made life in a mental hospital a never ending source of interest as it unfolded the inner lives of patients even in spite of our lack of ability to know how to get at the deeper facts. I developed during this time a number of specially interesting cases along the lines of research that I had learned with Sidis, and published a number of papers. I finally succeeded as the years went by in getting one promotion after another, so that while I began at the State Hospital as Fourth Assistant Physician, I ultimately arrived at the head of the medical staff as First Assistant Physician, which was the equivalent of Assistant Superintendent. The work of this position necessarily entailed additional administrative duties which were not altogether undesirable from my point of view, but with them all I never lost my personal contact with the patient and I still envy the ward physician his experiences of this sort. It was at this time, namely, 1903, when the opportunity came to make a trial for the Superintendency at Washington. This I did and succeeded, largely, I think, as a result of the quality of my interest and the work that I had done in the past. And so at the opening of the century I found myself again on a train alone and headed in a new direction with only the vaguest of ideas as to what lay at the other end of the journey.

# CHAPTER V

## SAINT ELIZABETHS

While it is true that I took the train for Washington without knowing what lay at the other end of the route, although I had visited Washington only a few months before and lectured on the Geographical Distribution of Insanity in the United States before the National Geographic Society and had there met my predecessor, whose sudden and unexpected death created the vacancy that I was going to fill, I did approach Washington with all the enthusiasm and great expectations of youth launched upon a great adventure. I had visions of the possibilities of the National Capital so far as I was concerned. I hoped that I would be able to carry on this new enterprise in the spirit of science, which had always been my ideal, and that I would be able to meet and personally contact men of ability in various scientific disciplines that were related in one way and another to psychiatry. In other words, I hoped to build up a scientifically conducted institution, scientifically backgrounded and with scientific ideals.

What I found, of course, was a practical problem which meant hard work and attention to details relating to a thousand different things that seemed to be very far remote from psychiatry. Saint Elizabeths Hospital had jogged along through the years at a comfortable pace, controlled and dominated by the humanitarian spirit. It had been brought into creation largely through the personal efforts of that marvelous product of American womanhood, Dorothea Lynde Dix, whose desk on which she is said to have written the Organic Act creating the hospital now stands in the Superintendent's quarters, and who during her lifetime had a room reserved for her use whenever she visited the hospital. The hospital's first Superintendent, Dr. Charles H. Nichols, was a Quaker, and the Quaker influence that came to us from England by way of the York Retreat was one of the outstanding features of its early years and left its distinct impression upon its traditions. During these years Dr. Pliny Earle, also a Quaker, used to visit the hospital frequently, and undoubtedly he also left the imprint of his ideas on the care of the " insane " upon the institution.

[28]

Without going into the history of Saint Elizabeths, I may only add that a little less than four years before I arrived on the scene Dr. A. B. Richardson had been appointed Superintendent, succeeding Dr. Godding, deceased. Dr. Richardson found an institution which with all of its kindly traditions had lagged somewhat behind on the construction side and had developed some rather quiet spots due to its then isolation, which had resulted, as they usually do, in a certain amount of stagnation. This is what happened to many of our hospitals during the transition period. They had been too conservative and had not quite kept up to what we now know would have been the most forward-looking standards. At any rate, the hospital was badly crowded, and Dr. Richardson being a new man, a personal appointment of President McKinley, was able almost at once to secure the then extraordinary sum of a million and a half dollars for construction. This included some twelve buildings for patients, a new administration building, a new kitchen building, and a new power house. When in the midst of the task he suddenly died, I came to Washington and inherited it. So that when I appeared upon the grounds all of this construction was under way, the grounds were in a condition that can be imaged with so many new buildings going up, and probably a thousand men were employed in this work. I had had very little experience in administration and I was pretty well overwhelmed by these new responsibilities, for in addition to seeing the construction work safely completed I had the task of readjusting the institution to the larger horizon which these new buildings and the extension of the hospital across Nichols Avenue to the other side of the road made necessary.

Aside from these technical conditions, I found certain parts of the institution in a rather primitive condition. The overcrowding had necessitated something like four hundred patients sleeping on the floor on straw mattresses, between which the night watchman made his rounds swinging on his arm an oil lantern. The wards for the untidy patients were tremendously crowded and understaffed, and despite the traditions that had come down from the past mechanical restraint in the form of camisoles and the bed saddle, which I had never before seen or heard of, were in use. This latter instrument was a steel frame in the form of a cross which was strapped to the bed, and the patient in turn was strapped to it, with outstretched hands strapped to its two arms. I am very happy to say that when I first saw this instrument I immediately issued an order prohibiting its further use, much to the discomfiture of all concerned, who, I am convinced, had a firm belief that it was impractical, if not impossible, to get along without it, nevertheless its abolition never produced any serious problems. I learned then and I know now that mechanical and chemical restraint, padded cells, strong rooms, and the like, are methods which are used for the purpose of avoiding the necessity of using one's brains, of thinking, of devising solutions and availing one's self of ingenuities and dexterities for overcoming difficulties. All of these things are much more difficult than to lock a patient up in a room, a method which I have long called systematic neglect. The abolition of the bed saddle and of all other forms of mechanical restraint forces the utilization of the brains of those who are responsible for the care of the patient, and results in the development of better methods, and in the long run, by a process of natural selection, it insures a better personnel.

In these early days, therefore, I was much immersed in getting acquainted with a really very complex institution and in learning my new duties as an administrative officer, how to make my contacts with the various government departments and officials, with Congress, and particularly with the Treasury Department, the auditors of which had a keen eye out for the mistakes of the new Superintendent. All of these matters were, however, in the course of time, negotiated successfully though not without a great amount of friction, a good many mistakes which the wisdom of later years would have prevented, and a Congressional investigation which provided front page literature for the Washington press for a considerable time. These, however, were necessary preliminaries. The physical plant of the hospital, its buildings and grounds, and particularly its power house, were all essential before questions of scientific care and management, innovations in treatment, and research work could even begin to function; and I soon came to feel this and not to resent the administrative duties as I saw many of my friends doing, but to learn that they were essential conditions precedent for the things that I hoped to accomplish. They provided the foundations, as it were, upon which the structure that I wanted to build must be erected. They created and kept in working order the conditions under which alone it was possible to do the work that I hoped to accomplish; and so I felt that my friends who thrashed around and complained about their administrative duties were really merely utilizing this particular excuse that lay handy as an alibi for doing nothing else. I early decided that this excuse might work with some people but that for me it was transparent and I would at least make the effort to continue my active interest in the scientific aspects of psychiatry.

I am constantly astonished in retrospect at my clarity of vision with regard to certain of these fundamental issues in those days, and it is one of the reasons why I have always respected the opinions of young people and have never felt that they should be minimized or that the young people themselves should be treated with condescension or in a patronizing manner. I have covered this point in my writings and have indicated that it may be that the younger people are the closer they are to the very sources of life and the truer they hew to the instinctive demands which lead in the right direction, and it is only as we get older that we accumulate prejudices and special interests which befog and distort the simple, straightforward issues of youth. However that may be, one of the most important things in these early days, an event that happened very shortly after my arrival in Washington in the fall of 1903, was to be asked by the Dean of the Medical Faculty of Georgetown University, Dr. George M. Kober, to accept the Professorship of Nervous and Mental Diseases and begin my lectures on neurology at once. I recognized this as an opportunity, and although I was very much overwhelmed at the burden of responsibility which was involved, I nevertheless accepted it and in due course started in. I remember the first lecture well. I was a pretty well scared young professor, and although I had prepared for this ordeal it was not an easy one. Dr. Kober, who in later years I counted one of my best friends, was present to see how the young professor showed up, and afterwards was most kindly in his enthusiastic comments on my efforts. During the next year, 1904, at the request of Dr. Emil A. de Schweinitz, Dean of the School of Medicine, I became Professor of Psychiatry of George Washington University.

It was with reference to these lectures that I had another of my clear insights into their significance for my future. I realized from the very beginning that in Washington, occupying the position I did, if I made a success of it I should probably be asked to speak or to lecture from time to time upon divers and sundry occasions, and that if I started in my lecture course for the students by writing out my lectures I would soon become a slave to the written page and would never acquire that spontaneity of utterance which is so much more valuable for the public speaker, both in retaining the interest and attention of his audience and in relieving him of the burdensome necessity of writing out everything in great detail for every occasion, to say nothing of the dampening effect it would have upon the development of any real spontaneity should he be called on unexpectedly to make a few remarks. And so from the very beginning I refused absolutely to do anything more than perhaps make a few pencil notes on a slip of paper; and week after week, and year after year, I gave these lectures, becoming, to be sure, progressively more comfortable in the situation but from time to time passing through moments when it seemed as if everything in the universe had come to an end, more particularly my own capacity for thinking. Standing before an audience with one's mouth open, as it were, to say the next sentence, and having every thought and every possibility of thinking disappear completely, effaced like the writing on a slate by a wet sponge, produces a sensation which, to put it mildly, is far from comfortable. But I fought my way through these disabilities, and I am glad that I was wise enough to foresee the desirability of this course.

It will be seen that in coming to Saint Elizabeths I had entered upon an exceedingly busy life, and although I had made every effort to prepare myself along the lines in which I had been least occupied, namely, various administrative aspects of the work, I found it very exacting. Aside from the very good sized job that I inherited from my predecessor, however, I also inherited disputes with certain doctors and lawyers and real estate representatives; and, as may be imagined, many of the employees of the Hospital, as well as salesmen, flocked to my office, trying to take advantage, I presume, of the newcomer who was not yet secure enough in his knowledge of his new position or experienced enough in the methods of meeting its difficulties. All of these matters gradually grew to proportions that resulted in a Congressional investigation which dragged out over a period of months with its public hearings, its newspaper notoriety, and all of the accompaniments which seem to be so dear to the news exploiting agencies and the American public. This experience was a difficult one, to be sure, but a very enlightening and broadening one, and contained more experience concentrated in a short space of time than I could have gathered over several years in any other way. It introduced me to the intricacies of legislative methods, the vicissitudes of public position, the necessities of self-control as well as of alertness; and it was an example, in rather large dimensions to be sure, of how Washington shakes down its newcomers. When the investigation was over I found myself pretty well tired out and that summer and the following four summers I took my vacation by going abroad.

# CHAPTER VI

## Europe—Military Psychiatry

As I stated at the end of the last chapter, following the Congressional investigation of the Hospital I went to Europe for my vacation and I followed this practice in all for five consecutive years.

The immediate objective of my first trip was the French Neurological Congress at Lille, which I attended, incidentally meeting a number of well known and prominent neurologists and psychiatrists of the Continent. Subsequently I attended the First International Congress of Psychiatry, Neurology and Psychology and the Care of the Insane, at Amsterdam, in September, 1907, and the Third International Congress for the Care of the Insane in Vienna in October, 1908. On all of these occasions I met the prominent people of the world in my specialty. I have always believed that the greatest benefit that we attain from attending medical society meetings is our personal contacts. These give us an opportunity to size up people whose works we have read and whom we have read about, and we get opinions as a result that cannot be obtained in any other way and which I believe to be invaluable. At the end of this period, therefore, it will be seen that I had met personally a very considerable percentage of the outstanding neurologists and psychiatrists of Europe, as these Congresses were especially well attended. At Amsterdam I met Professor Carl G. Jung for the first time, and at Vienna I attended the unveiling of the bust of Professor R. von Krafft-Ebing at the University and the subsequent induction into office of Professor Wagner von Jauregg, who in later years was responsible for the introduction of the malaria therapy for paresis and who has recently retired from his professorship.

In the meantime I traveled pretty well over the Continent and visited a large number of institutions for the care of the "insane," and in some instances other types of hospitals. I could tell many interesting stories about my wanderings, but for the most part they would have very little point for the present purposes. My mind in these days was acquisitive. I saw, I took in, I was curious and interested, but I had found no satisfactory pathway through all these

discrete facts. No fundamental principles seemed to stand out. I
saw institutions of all kinds and descriptions, good, bad, and indifferent, progressive and hopeless. I saw restraint in all its crudity. I
remember one institution which I visited where, when I entered one
of the wards occupied by some forty men, I found every one of them
stark naked and strapped to his bed. There was only one bed that
was not occupied by a patient and that was occupied by a giant of
an attendant who was asleep. He jumped up as we came in and
walked through the ward with us, and I remember these naked men
cursing us and spitting at us as we went by. No more lurid example
of the evils of restraint has ever come to my attention, and the picture
of this scene remains indelibly impressed upon my mind. I learned
incidentally that of the staff of physicians who ran this institution of
some twelve or fourteen hundred beds—I have forgotten just how
many—only one was on duty at a time and he spent most of his time
in the laboratory. Therefore if the institution can be said to have
run at all it ran itself, and this was the result, the result that is usually
found under such circumstances. A hospital as a rule cannot maintain itself for any length of time at a level superior to its superintendent. His ideals seep down through all the various levels of the
institution, and the institution, if he has been there any length of
time, represents him. It is very important, therefore, that the superintendent should have ideals that are definite and to which he can
hew year in and year out, for continuity of application and direction
and clear-cut purpose are essential to establishing adequate standards
and afterwards to maintaining them.

The final year and the fifth I spent at Munich, taking the six
weeks' extension course which was given at the Psychiatric Clinic,
then conducted by Professor Kraepelin. This was an intensive
course in psychiatry and its various allied subjects to which eminent
men from other cities were invited to contribute. The course consisted of lectures, clinics, and demonstrations beginning in the morning, I think at nine o'clock, and lasting straight through until about
five or six o'clock in the afternoon, with an occasional trip to another
institution or a supper together to get acquainted. The class consisted of in the neighborhood of forty or fifty students that came from
all parts of the world. And so here was another broadening and
decidedly helpful experience. We came under the influence of
Kraepelin's dynamic and stimulating personality and the admirable
teaching of his associates, particularly Professor Alois Alzheimer,

who then was the outstanding histopathologist of the nervous system in the world, and Professor Felix Plaut, who had done so much to put the Wassermann reaction on the map.   Then there was Professor Kobinian Brodmann with his fascinating lectures on the comparative morphology of the brain cortex, and Professor C. von Monakow, head of the Anatomical Institute at Zurich, who lectured to us on the nervous system, particularly the results of some of his own researches. He had then only recently formulated his theory of diaschisis.

It is one of my most pleasant memories to recall that Professor Kraepelin with Professor Plaut visited this country the summer before Professor Kraepelin died and that they spent in the neighborhood of two weeks in Washington, much of the time at Saint Elizabeths.   Professor Kraepelin was studying particularly the negro, for he had always been interested in comparative psychiatry and he was especially interested in the reaction of the negro to syphilis.   This was a delightful renewal of a friendship with my old Professor, who I found at seventy years of age had just the same keen, alert mind and active interest in psychiatry that he had had all through his life.

I came back from these European trips with a great deal of detailed information and a great deal of scientific enthusiasm, especially as a result of my Munich experience.   When it came to applying this enthusiasm and this information to the immediate matters of administration it became necessary to clarify my ideas considerably and this process of clarification has been going on slowly through the years.   For instance, I have been interested consistently to develop scientific work, and I think Saint Elizabeths Hospital has turned out its share.   But when I think of all of the institutions of Europe that I laboriously and systematically examined I think of a group of foreign editions of what I was already familiar with in this country— ward after ward in institutions, some of which were clean and some of which were dirty, some well managed, some poorly managed, some using restraint freely and others not, some well built and planned and others poorly and cheaply built, but the patients in all of them, no matter what their nationality, looking very much alike, acting very much alike, and apparently responding to their various kinds of care very much in the same way as we were accustomed to see them here.

I did bring over to the new buildings some ideas of decoration and some pictures to hang upon the walls.   But perhaps the principal thing that I brought in those early days was the concept of military psychiatry.   I noticed particularly at Heidelberg the classes of Army officers, and in Berlin, at the Charité, that Professor Theodor Ziehen spent much of his time teaching medical officers of the Army, and in other places I saw evidences of the same thing. I thought this through as best I could and suggested to the then Surgeon General of the Army, Dr. George H. Torney, that the Army Medical Corps establish a liaison with Saint Elizabeths Hospital for the purpose of gaining experience in psychiatry and with the added objective of military psychiatry. Dr. Torney fortunately had an open mind to this proposition as his son, who happened to be a friend of mine, was a psychiatrist in the New York State Hospital Service. I had observed the great wastage in military forces of taking in defective youths and attempting to make soldiers of them, and I suggested this method in order to devise a more efficient and economic way of dealing with military personnel. This was the beginning of what has been followed out through the years, namely, systematic instruction and experience in psychiatry, not only in the Army but in the Navy and the Public Health Service, so that now both branches of the military establishment have psychotic wards and men who have had considerable experience in dealing with mental disease. The necessity for military psychiatry and its worthwhileness was disclosed later in the Russo-Japanese War. In the early days of our entry into the World War I had the pleasure and honor of introducing to the then Surgeon General of the Army, General William C. Gorgas, a group of psychiatrists who came with a proposition to erect a psychiatric unit in connection with a military hospital and had the money already in hand to cover the expenses of its construction. This money, $15,000 I believe was the amount, was donated by Miss Anne Thompson, of Philadelphia, and after the War was over we had the pleasure of giving to Miss Thompson the flag that flew over this unit. This was the beginning of the psychiatric service in our forces during this great conflict.

My European travels, then, were exceedingly valuable not only as orientation experiences but as stimulating from many points of view. I made many personal contacts which have maintained through the years, and acquired information and experience which formed an invaluable background for further development.

# CHAPTER VII

## DEVELOPMENTS

It will be remembered that during my connection with the New York State Service I had spent some time at the Pathological Institute, working more particularly with Dr. Sidis upon certain problems of what we called in those days mental dissociation. In 1899 the Medico-Psychological Association had its annual meeting in New York and one of its sessions was held at the Pathological Institute, which was housed in the Metropolitan Life Building, No. 1 Madison Avenue. On this occasion by invitation I read my first paper before this organization, for I had not yet become a member and did not join it until 1902. It is my recollection that it was at this meeting that I first met Mr. Adolf Meyer and Dr. August Hoch, with both of whom I was to be later more or less closely associated over a considerable period of years.

During these early contacts with the Medico-Psychological Association I heard much about the Annual Address that had been given at the Philadelphia meeting in 1894 by Dr. S. Weir Mitchell,* the grand old man of neurology of those days. Dr. Mitchell in his address took the members of the Association roundly to task for their isolation from the rest of the profession and their failure to contribute to the scientific progress of their specialty, and he drew the picture of an ideal hospital for mental disease presided over by a neurologist who was interested solely in the medical problems and who because of his broad interest and his contributions to research would be a constant source of stimulus to the medical staff. He felt that the then ninety-one thousand " insane " being cared for by members of the Association ought to result in marked contributions to scientific medicine, but that the superintendents were content to drift along without contact with the rest of the profession, without stimulus from the outside world, as the administrative officers of large caravansaries where the principal problems were feeding, clothing, housing and building. The physician in charge of the hospital should be relieved from all executive duties by a steward who takes care of

---

* Mitchell, S. Weir: Address before the 50th Annual Meeting American Medico-Psychological Association, May, 1894. Proceedings Amer. Medico-Psychological Ass'n, Vol. I, 1894, p. 101.

those things for him—and he painted a picture of the hospital more like those with which he was accustomed to personally deal.   This address, while Dr. Mitchell was very apologetic for its critical tone, was accepted by the members of the Association in an extraordinarily kindly way.   They rather felt the shortcomings that they were accused of and yet, I suspect, hardly knew how to extricate themselves from the dilemma into which his argument had plunged them. His address was answered in a succeeding number of the *American Journal of Insanity* by Dr. Walter Channing,* who came forward boldly in defense of the superintendents, showed very clearly their limitations and that their main duties had of necessity been and continued to be the providing for the ever-increasing number of mentally ill, decent living conditions, and that until this could be done it was hardly to be expected that developments along the line Dr. Mitchell suggested would be possible.

I pondered these matters considerably in those days.   Many years later, in 1925, when I became President of the Association, which had by that time changed its name to the American Psychiatric Association, I devoted part of my Presidential Address† to a defense of the superintendents of these early days, in the following words:

"Before going on to a discussion of some of the more vital present-day issues of psychiatry I feel impelled to pause by the way, as it were, and to pay tribute to the hospital superintendents of one and two generations ago.   I do this perhaps out of a certain sense of guilt, because I am afraid that during the period of my psychiatric adolescence I may have joined in my feelings with certain others at the same stage of development and made fun of these sturdy gentlemen because they published annual reports of state hospitals in which were pictured the prize pumpkin at the county fair and the tallest corn raised in the state.   I wish now to make amends for a state of mind the only excuse for which was ignorance and lack of experience.

"The old-fashioned hospital superintendent, if I may call him that, using the qualification as an endearment rather than as a criticism, we must remember was on the firing line in those stormy days when he was trying to rescue the 'insane' from the ignorance, the stupidity, the superstition and the cruelty of the times.   He was animated by an understanding of these unfortunate people that was born of a humanitarian instinct and that

---

* Channing, Walter: Some Remarks on the Address Delivered to the American Medico-Psychological Association, by S. Weir Mitchell, M.D., May 16, 1894.  Amer. Journal of Insanity, Vol. 51, Oct., 1894, p. 171.
† White, W. A.:  Presidential Address.  American Journal of Psychiatry, Vol. 5, No. 1, July, 1925, p. 1.

he was for the most part, I suspect, quite incapable of formulating in any academic phraseology. He felt, and he knew because he felt, that the existing state of affairs was wrong and indefensible, and he saw with what we must acknowledge at this time was marvelous clearness the direction in which the remedy lay, and what is more important than all he had the courage and the strength of purpose to put his program through. We youngsters who came along a generation after the main victories in this fight had been won knew little of this past history and were inclined to criticize the old-fashioned superintendent because he did not have a scientific interest in psychiatry nor a scientific vision. We did not appreciate that at the time when his services were most valuable if he did not have scientific information about psychiatry there was a very good reason for his lack, because there was no scientific information in existence. We did not appreciate as we must now that even if there had been what we might properly call a scientific psychiatry in existence science alone would never have rescued the ' insane ' from the superstition of the times and would never have created the state hospital.

" The pumpkin and the corn in the annual report are symbolic, perhaps, of the simple, uncomplicated, and, if you will, unscientific thinking of the old-fashioned superintendent. He believed in taking the mentally ill into the hospital just about as you would take an individual into your family and in making the hospital as far as possible a home-like institution with all of the homely traditions and virtues and occupations, and so he built his hospital along these lines. He conducted it like a large family of which he was the father. He undertook to know each patient and each employee personally, and he believed that the hospital should not grow in size beyond the point where this personal contact was possible. He believed in teaching the simple occupations, particularly farming, for he believed in getting close to nature, in working outdoors in the sunlight and the fresh air, in raising the food that was to be eaten; and in commenting upon these various ideals I cannot but wonder in passing whether our very intelligent college graduates who have come into the hospital under the designation of occupational therapists have added very much that is of value to these original conceptions. They have the information and the training which should make them able to add much of value, but whether they have the traditions and the background which will direct this information and training into the most valuable lines remains to be seen. I think they undoubtedly will do this in time; perhaps they already have. At any rate occupational training has had a very interesting past, and I have no doubt it will have a very interesting future.

" Perhaps the most valuable thing from our point of view that the old superintendent did was to create the state hospital, because after all the state hospital as it stands today is the very foundation of psychiatry. That foundation was well built, it was splendidly conceived, its traditions and its ideals are all that could be wished for, and it is because of the old superintendent's vision and courage and humanitarian instincts that this is true; and if today we are able to build a scientific psychiatry, as we believe we are doing, it is largely due to the fact that we have had this firm foundation upon which to raise our superstructure."

While there was much that was stimulating and thought-provoking in Dr. Mitchell's address, it was obvious that he did not understand the situation from the inside, as it were, and that while he personally with his dominant, kindly, and intellectually high-geared personality might have wrought wonders with many of the patients, that merely to go through certain routines of pupillary examinations, testing knee jerks, etc., has very little to do with either scientific medicine or research. It became essential first to establish the state hospital as a going concern, with the major problems of construction and supplies and administration sufficiently worked out so as not to be stumbled over at every turn. It needed to be understood that the superintendent had to be a physician, not any physician but a physician well informed in the specialty of mental disease. The double-headed management had been tried and wherever tried it had failed, unless, as occasionally happened, the two heads were closely related on the basis of personal friendship. As I saw it, every problem of a great hospital that undertakes not only the care and treatment of acute illness but takes over the whole problem of the regulation of the lives of its patients for years at a time is a medical problem, whether it be merely the question of whether there should be bars at the window, or whether hydrotherapy shall be used and what for and how, whether or not there shall be a farm or a dairy, what particular type of machine for any particular purpose is preferable— every question in fact, because every question has to do with the environment and the lives of the patients and therefore becomes directly of medical significance. These great hospitals had of necessity to grow up and be organized and administered by men who were interested in these aspects of the environment, and interested in this specific way; and not only that, but inasmuch as there can not be two captains to a ship these duties of purchasing and administering the personnel and the medical needs must have a certain amount of medical supervision and direction if they are to fit into the general picture, and, more important in a practical way, if the superintendent is actually to be held responsible for the administration of the hospital. If he is, then his powers and duties must be commensurate with his responsibilities.

I began to see the situation in this light quite early and I saw in addition that the concept of a superintendent from this point of view was not by any means altogether discouraging: that whereas the superintendent himself might not be able to conduct personal research and to be engaged professionally in the care of patients, he could make his life much more useful than if he were, by organizing a plan and creating a situation in which twenty, fifty or a hundred men might have an opportunity to do all of these things that he had to relinquish. And so really his position as superintendent gave him a glorious opportunity for affording the means wherewith the work that Dr. Mitchell was quite anxious to see the superintendent do personally could probably be better done by the men who took his place, some of whom at least might be privileged to be relieved of administrative duties entirely and to devote themselves exclusively to scientic work. This was a concept which satisfactorily replaced the other, and I found myself working enthusiastically to these ends, also quite conscious of the fact, as I have already indicated, that the cry of not having time to do this, that or the other thing is generally an alibi. Often, I have no doubt, the superintendent in many institutions has plenty of time to work in the laboratory if he so desired. I usually find in my experience that the things people want to do they somehow find time to do. If there is any excuse on the basis of time for lack of accomplishment so far as the superintendent and the medical officers are concerned, it is not due strictly to lack of time but to lack of ability to control the distribution of time; for after all, although we are all public officers and although we may elect to spend an hour or two in the afternoon in meditation over a microscope the world of duty is all too apt to break in upon that time and command our presence and our thought. However, the principle as I have laid it down is fairly clear, and it will be developed in various directions as we proceed.

Dr. Mitchell in his address in setting forth what he conceived to be an ideal institution developed it along the lines that we speak of now as the " cottage plan." In my trips through Europe I had found institutions, especially the newer ones, built along these lines. The old type of hospital where all of the patients were supposed to be housed in a single building, which was the original plan upon which our state hospitals were constructed, gradually gave way in various directions until finally the so-called cottage plan was the type of institution that took its place. My predecessor, Dr. Richardson, had devised the extensions for Saint Elizabeths Hospital along these lines, and the buildings which I found under construction when I came here varied in size, accommodating at the minimum thirty-five or forty patients and at the maximum one hundred and twenty odd. In such institutions as Egelfing, which is the hospital that Kraepelin built just outside of Munich, this cottage plan was carried out very beautifully. The cottages were quite small. It would seem to me that they could not have accommodated over twenty patients, as I recall it. They were built of different designs and harmoniously grouped so that the hospital looked very much like a modern real estate subdivision which was being developed. This very attractive way of building an institution appealed to me not only because of its attractiveness, which in itself is an important asset, but because of the possibility of a much more satisfactory grouping of patients which this plan provides. And so in the later developments that I have had the privilege of superintending at Saint Elizabeths we have continued to build separate buildings for separate types of patients, much larger than twenty-bed cottages, to be sure, but the principle involved is the same nevertheless.

After my experience in Munich I was very much impressed with the desirability of the psychopathic hospital, or, as I advocated more particularly later on, of the psychopathic pavilion in connection with the general hospital. The Institute at Munich was only one of such hospitals in Germany to which acute patients were brought and kept for varying periods of time and then, provided they did not get well, transferred to what would correspond in our country to the state hospital. It was constructed and equipped in every way for the most careful and detailed scientific research and highly specialized medical care, and in addition its large lecture room was utilized for teaching purposes. There not only did the students from the medical school come for their clinical lectures, but the students from the law school also; and as I saw the Institute fitting into the general life of the city of Munich, so that its police for example were instructed to bring persons who had attempted suicide immediately to the clinic rather than to the police station, I felt the great significance of such an institution in our American municipality. We had already made a start in this direction in Albany, where Pavilion F, as it was called, of the Albany Hospital, was devoted to the care of mental cases under the direction of Dr. J. Montgomery Mosher. This scheme worked so well that subsequent developments began to take the form in this country that they had already assumed abroad, and the Boston Psychopathic Hospital as one of the teaching units of the Harvard Medical School, and the Phipps Psychiatric Clinic as one of the pavilions of the Johns Hopkins Hospital, were the earliest developments in this direction. Others have followed. Here in Washington there was a municipal hospital, so-called Washington Asylum and Jail, which in these early days was rather a disgrace to the city than something to be proud of. Its buildings were of wood, terrible fire risks, overcrowded, incapable of adequate sanitation, and quite in line with poorhouse construction of the nineteenth century. Nevertheless there was a ward set apart for the mental cases, and as primitive as it was, it was the psychopathic ward. In later years when the city of Washington decided to rebuild its municipal hospital in accordance with modern standards of hospital construction I am pleased to record that the psychopathic pavilion was the first unit built. The name of the institution is now Gallinger Municipal Hospital.

Psychopathic pavilions which stand by themselves have disadvantages as well as advantages. They are reception hospitals for the acutely psychotic patient and almost invariably they soon become so crowded that the principal job of the medical staff is to get patients out so that they will have room to take others in. It thus becomes a wild race against time to keep the population moving. Under these circumstances the careful and deliberate study and treatment of acute illness is not possible, and, which is also very unfortunate, the medical staff never see the patient except for the few days that he is in the pavilion and so they are not at all acquainted in their experience with the course of mental illness over a long period of time and with its forms of termination. If such hospitals could be maintained at a high standard of scientific and therapeutic excellence without having to deal with this everlasting problem of admission and discharge they would be much more useful. But in any case their maximum usefulness is attained when they are attached to a medical center and thus become on the one hand a part of a great general hospital and on the other a part of a great medical school, so that they can be used for teaching purposes in the latter instance; and as a result of the alliance with the general hospital the medical internes may be rotated through the psychopathic pavilion and the medical staff of the pavilion may be used for consultation on the general medical wards, thus tying up psychiatry with general medicine in some such way as, I suspect, Dr. Mitchell had in mind.

It is interesting to note that development is taking place in just these ways.  General hospitals are putting in wards for the care of mental cases, medical centers are including the psychopathic department, and great centers of medical education are utilizing these opportunities.  They are being utilized because they are being found to work to the advantage of all concerned.  The psychiatrist is enlarging his horizon by his contact with general medicine, and the general practitioner and the medical specialist are learning some of the fundamentals of psychiatric practice.  And now the latest development that is happening at the present moment is the modification of the medical curriculum to include a reasonable number of hours devoted to the study of the mind and its disorders.  When it is appreciated that 50 per cent of the beds in the hospitals of the United States are occupied by mental cases, it does not seem too much to expect that the medical schools should occupy themselves to some extent with equipping their graduates to deal with this numerically and economically very important group of maladies.

# CHAPTER VIII

## The Beginning of the Century

As I have already indicated and as must be patent to anyone trying to visualize the situation, an account of the care of the " insane " in the United States can not be pursued in a systematic, chronological manner, and, as the reader will have already discovered, I have not undertaken to do so. Progress took place at very different rates in different states, and in some states it did not seem to take place at all over long periods. Therefore my description is what might be called a functional description, which I will undertake to relate to the time factor only incidentally.

The state of the care of the " insane " at the beginning of this century might therefore, from what has already been said, be summed up in some such fashion as this: The state hospital had come into existence very definitely as the solution of the economic and political problems involved. It had been slowly coming to be appreciated that counties and municipalities, unless they were large ones, were too small political subdivisions to undertake the economic burden of the care of the " insane." It was a problem that could be assumed only by the State. This idea fitted in with what was happening from another angle, namely, the coming into being and the development of the humanitarian period in the history of this care. This, of course, is roughly dated from Pinel's release of the " insane " at the Salpêtrière in 1793, but the significance of this act of Pinel took a long time to gain recognition, and of course in many instances a long time to even be heard of. But the attitude toward the mentally ill which this act of Pinel symbolizes did finally become the moving principle at the foundation of the major changes in their care and treatment which took place during the latter part of the nineteenth century in this country, largely under the inspirational guidance of Dorothea Lynde Dix, and the impetus of which was carried on into the twentieth century. And so the acceptance of the care of the " insane " as a problem properly belonging to the state fitted in with the humanitarian movement which was directed to removing the " insane " from the almshouses and the jails where so many hundreds of them were kept confined in the most deplorable state of neglect

and misery. This movement, of course, even yet has not reached its
final stage of development; but in these early days it was a God-send
to these afflicted people to be covered into the great state hospitals,
imperfect from a medical and scientific point of view as these institutions admittedly were. But one can not think of these imperfec-
tions without realizing, as Dr. Channing well said in his answer to
Dr. Mitchell, that the main problem of these days was, after all, this
great humanitarian problem, and I might add to that commentary the
fact that there was not very much known about mental medicine
anyway by anybody. It was all more or less a region of mystery, and
good intentions and intuition and tact were probably the most
valuable instruments that we possessed for handling our human
problems.

In the early days of the state hospital, in New York State, for
example, there had been a distinction between the acutely and the
chronically ill. The Utica State Hospital was originally built to take
in the acute types of cases. Even in those early days a single hospital
could hardly expect to take care of the mentally ill in a great state
like New York, and so this natural distinction was made. The
patients went there with the prospect of getting well, and when the
load became so great as to be beyond the capacity of Utica to care
for it, other state hospitals were built and at first they were built
wholly for the chronic " insane." And so we had, for example, a
hospital like the Willard State Hospital designated as the Willard
State Hospital for the Chronic Insane. It soon became obvious that
such a distinction, while it might have some advantages, had many
drawbacks, and to take a patient to an institution where he found in
any direction that he looked the label which indicated that he was in
an institution for the chronic " insane " was hardly an experience
that could be calculated to stimulate him on the road to recovery. So
as the hospitals multiplied the practice grew up of expecting each
hospital to take all of the mental cases in a certain designated group
of counties surrounding it, so that each institution, so to speak, was
responsible within its own zone of influence. This worked out better,
for not only was the institution for the chronic " insane " a discouraging institution to which to send a patient but it was also a
discouraging institution from which to expect anything, medical or
scientific results, or anything else. The name alone was sufficient to
destroy all initiative.

Nevertheless the need of institutions in the large metropolitan
districts to which patients might be sent pending their transfer to the

great state hospitals, which for the most part occupied territory far removed from these centers of population, became more and more obvious. This need was met by the psychopathic pavilion such as existed for so many years in Bellevue Hospital, to which patients were admitted pending their examination, commitment and transfer to the great hospital on Ward's Island. The first of these psychopathic pavilions was Pavilion F in connection with the Albany Hospital, which came into existence technically in 1899 but which opened for its first admission February 18, 1902. As I have already stated, this plan has now been followed by many cities, and the psychopathic pavilion or the psychopathic ward in the general hospital is now an established institution, although with certain drawbacks that I have already mentioned. To these I might add, perhaps, that it, like its predecessor, the institution for the care of only acute cases, somewhat tends to perpetuate the distinction between the acute and the chronic, but this is not as a rule such a serious matter with these institutions because all patients have to be discharged within a comparatively short time, as new ones are continually coming in.

Along with these developments came the principle of non-restraint, so ably set forth and supported by Dr. Charles W. Page, for many years Superintendent of Danvers State Hospital, Massachusetts, who in turn had received his inspiration largely from Dr. John Connolly, Superintendent of the asylum at Hanwell, England. The principle of non-restraint was accepted and received lip worship, at least, pretty generally, although like all such radical modifications it was slow of acceptance because slow to be understood. The fact of the matter was that those who for years had automatically applied camisoles to disturbed patients did not know how to do anything else. When a patient became violent and irritated and fighting they knew nothing better than to tie him up. They did not realize, as was emphasized over and over again, that in the institution where mechanical restraint did not exist such conditions as I have briefly indicated did not develop, and even if they did understand it they did not know how to make the transition. So it is not strange, perhaps, that this principle of non-restraint was so slow in being translated into practical performance. It is only a little while ago that I visited one of our supposedly well conducted hospitals and saw a whole group of men on one ward laced up in camisoles. I could hardly believe my eyes, but there it was in a hospital that had no dearth of personnel, no lack of money, to excuse it, but only lack of experience and of understanding. And it was only a few months

ago that a superintendent of a great institution for the care of the
" insane " visited us and after he had been taken through a number
of wards he asked to be taken through our worst wards, where the
patients were violent, and when he was told that he had already been
through those wards he showed very clearly not only his surprise but,
I fear, his incredulity.  In other words, he could hardly believe that
we were telling him the exact truth.  From his point of view there
must have been a joker in the situation somewhere.  And yet this
experience happened right here within the year.

It will be remembered that one of my first acts when I came to
Saint Elizabeths was to order the abolition of the form of restraint
known as the saddle.  I merely wish to add at this point that I have
never ceased to bear this matter of restraint in mind and to consider
it in its ramifications in every direction.  One must think of it not
only in terms of camisoles and strong sheets and wristlets, and the
like, but in terms of those restraining influences in the environment
which are repressive in nature.  Repressive personalities, for
example, can be as destructive as physical agencies, perhaps more so.
In considering, therefore, all the problems of construction, the aim
is as far as possible to develop institutions that are as unlike the old
asylum as they can be made.  As I often put it, in the old asylum
if the patient threw a chair across the room they screwed the chair
to the floor, if he broke out a window-pane they covered the window
with a heavy screen, if he struck somebody in the face they handcuffed him, etc., etc.—each act of expression was followed by an
act equal and in the opposite direction of repression—of restraint, and
restraint means not only restraint but in addition it always means
frustration and as frustration it is always bad.  So we are gradually
developing in the direction not only of lack of restraint in the usual
meaning of that term but of the construction of a hospital environment which will be as little repressive as possible, and then, beyond
that, which will invite the patient out into creative activities.  This
relation of the environment to the patient is a very important one.
It is one that is ordinarily given little consideration, and it is
obviously one that Dr. Mitchell had not really sensed when he wrote
his criticism, for, after all, even the old asylums did take the patient
out of the environment in which he had developed his psychosis and
where the forces operated that produced this result.

One of the difficulties that resulted from the efforts at abolishing
mechanical restraint was its replacement by the use of sedative and
narcotic drugs, the use of which came to be called, very appropri-

ately, " chemical restraint." I have already referred to this and I can only say at this point, in addition to what I have already said, that this class of drugs practically need not be used at all in a great hospital for mental diseases except from time to time in an emergency. Their constant and daily use produces delirioid reactions such as I have already described and actually, like mechanical restraint, creates the very conditions it is designed to cure. Chemical restraint, like mechanical restraint, at the opening of the century was falling into disrepute, slowly, of course, as is the tempo of all such movements, but, I verily believe, surely.

One of the developments which came in with the century and which has helped very markedly to minimize the use of mechanical and chemical restraint was the development of hydrotherapy. The use of water in one way or another in the treatment of the mentally ill, particularly those that were acutely disturbed, seemed to make an immediate appeal to hospital managements everywhere, with the result that it came to be largely used for patients who otherwise would have been physically restrained or chemically restrained. It is, of course, somewhat unfortunate, but apparently inevitable, that in certain stages it became a substitute for such restraint, and the wet pack as applied was really a form of mechanical restraint, to which, of course, was added the soothing effect of warmth and, what is much more important, the continuous personal care and supervision of a bath attendant or a nurse. Hydrotherapeutic measures developed not only along these lines but along the lines which were contemporaneously developing in Europe, namely, the use of the continuous bath. In Europe the patient was placed in the bath and sometimes stayed there for weeks or months at a time. That practice has rarely been followed in this country but patients are put in the continuous bath for a number of hours, and the sedative effect of the warm water is far superior to the sedation that is produced by drugs. Here, too, in the earlier days there was a tendency to make the continuous bath a form of restraint by strapping a sheet across the top of the tub, but with a number of accidents that followed as a result of this practice the tendency is for it to disappear.

I have already indicated the advantages of the cottage plan of construction. At the opening of the century this plan was much in favor and came to be very generally adopted as the best method of development, for reasons already indicated, of a large institution for mental disease; so that at the present time most of our large hospitals, or at least those portions of them that have been constructed within the last few years, have been developed in accordance with this plan.

Another development which came in with the century, although of course it had scattered beginnings before that, was the utilization of trained personnel, which was more especially brought to pass by the development in the hospital of its own training school for nurses. This movement had so many things to recommend it that when instituted in any institution it was there to stay, so that most of the large state hospitals have their own training schools and many of the larger or better endowed private institutions have also. This was the beginning of a widespread movement to train the personnel of the hospital in their duties, to educate them in what was expected of them, to teach them how they must needs coöperate in a large and complicated plan which focused upon the welfare of the patient. Such trained personnel inevitably raised the standard of care. Not only was the care more intelligent but it became more personal and highly individualized. Although the early efforts to imitate the general hospital by treating the patients as if they were physically ill and so keeping them in bed, taking their temperatures, making all sorts of physical examinations on the theory that there was something to be found that might account for the mental disorder, did not get very far from this point of view, it did raise the standard of care decidedly and it did increase the interest in the patient from a purely medical point of view. So that while not much resulted in the way of curing patients of mental disease by putting them through this sort of procedure, still here were certain things to take hold of for future development. Then, of course, the existence of the training school required the staff to do systematic teaching, which was an added incentive to them to keep their information clear-cut, well formulated and readily available.

In addition to all of this and going along at the same time was the gradual acceptance and understanding of Kraepelin's contribution to the description of the psychoses. His delimitation of the two great groups, the manic-depressive and the dementia precox groups, threw a great ray of light into this region where before there had been little else than confusion and darkness. It is very hard for the physician who practices in one of these great institutions today to appreciate how little a physician of forty years ago had to work with. This Kraepelinian contribution was of inestimable benefit to everyone connected with the patient.

In the old days of forty years ago there was no trained personnel, there was no hydrotherapy, there was no scientific understanding of mental disorder, there was no recognized medical procedure except to temporize with periods of excitement and to watch those patients who were suicidal. There were no stimulating contacts with other physicians or with the outside world, and therefore there was very little upon which anyone short of a genius could build. Then at the opening of the century, a date which I fixed arbitrarily for purposes of convenience, all these various lines of development converged to the same end, namely, the welfare of the patient; and we can see what an impetus was given all along the line to the development of the care and the treatment of mental disease. Perhaps I should mention one tool which the old state hospital used then and which the state hospital uses now to very great advantage, and that is employment. This is particularly a well used tool in those institutions that are located in country districts, drawing their populations from agricultural regions, where the main activities of the hospital are the conduct of a large farm supplying food for the patient population. Here we have one of the most wholesome of all therapeutic agencies, healthy outdoor work, normal physical fatigue; and this sort of work, I am afraid, has never been improved upon. But it will be seen, even with this advantage, how meager were the opportunities in these early days. The hospitals even lacked an appropriate place to perform a surgical operation if the emergency arose. The amputation of a gangrenous leg, which occasionally had to be done, had to be accomplished in an ordinary room prepared especially for that purpose and an outside surgeon called in to do it. Under such circumstances surgical procedures were rarely resorted to. The same may be said of dental procedures, the care of the eye, etc. Everything in these great institutions had been subordinated to the great humanitarian endeavor of getting patients out of the miserable and sordid surroundings of jails and poorhouses and into decently clean, physically comfortable institutions where they could have plenty of good wholesome food and the opportunity of work in the open air on a farm; and until this was accomplished development along these various other lines had to remain waiting.

# CHAPTER IX

## The Value of an Idea—Psychoanalysis

The last chapter describes briefly the stage of development to which the care of the " insane " had arrived during the first years of the century. Other things happened beyond those that are mentioned in that chapter. As already indicated, the acceptance of the Kraepelinian system of classification and description of the course and outcome of the psychoses had a tremendously stimulating effect all along the line. Psychiatry, mental medicine, psychopathology, were coming to be special disciplines in fact rather than in name only; and investigations in these various departments took on more and more the flavor of scientific methods, and everyone connected with the care of the " insane " felt that somehow he was more organically related to the general practice of medicine and more respectably attuned to the harmonies of scientific progress than he had ever been before. The influence of Kraepelin was really tremendous, not only in America but all over the world. He raised what might be called descriptive psychiatry to the highest peak it had ever attained.

With asylums having changed to hospitals, and with the hospitals having become hospitals in fact instead of in name only, with the recognition of the scientific ramifications of mental medicine, with the acceptance pretty generally of the application of the general principles of medicine so far as they were needed, with the installation in a number of hospitals of laboratories not only for general clinical work but which were expected to turn out also research work, with the insistence upon autopsies and the introduction of the microscope,— the complexion of the old asylum was indeed changing very radically in many directions. To be sure, the changes had been slow, but they were sure, and in each instance, backed up by experience, they were generally accepted. So growth and development went along lines which became fairly well established. The Medico-Psychological Association* appointed its committees on training schools, on research,

* The American Medico-Psychological Association was originally the Association of Medical Superintendents of American Institutions for the Insane and its name was changed from this to American Medico-Psychological Association in 1892, while in 1921 the name was again changed to the American Psychiatric Association, the name which it at present bears.

etc., and finally they made a very valuable study which resulted in the setting up of the minimum standards required for a hospital for the " insane," as outlined by the Committee on Standards and Policies and presented at the eightieth annual meeting of the American Psychiatric Association in 1924 and revised at the meeting the following year.* It is well to quote these standards at this point. They are as follows:

" 1. The chief executive officer must be a well qualified physician and experienced psychiatrist whose appointment and removal shall not be controlled by partisan politics.

2. All other persons employed at the institution ought to be subordinate to him and subject to removal by him if they fail to discharge their duties properly.

3. The positions and administration of the institution must be free from control for the purposes of partisan politics.

4. There must be an adequate medical staff of well qualified physicians; the proportion to total patients to be not less than 1 to 150 in addition to the superintendent, and to the number of patients admitted annually not less than 1 to 40. There must be one or more full-time dentists.

5. There must be a staff of consulting specialists at least in internal medicine, general surgery, organic neurology, diseases of the eye, ear, nose and throat, and radiology, employed under such terms as will ensure adequate services. A record of their visits must be kept.

6. The medical staff must be organized, the services well defined and the clinical work under the direction of a staff leader or clinical director.

7. Each medical service must be provided with an office and an examining room, containing suitable conveniences and equipment for the work to be performed, and with such clerical help specially assigned to the service as may be required for the keeping of the medical and administrative records.

8. There must be carefully kept clinical histories of all the patients, in proper files for ready reference on each service.

9. Statistical data relating to each patient must be recorded in accordance with the standards system adopted by the Association.

10. The patients must be classified in accordance with their mental and physical condition, with adequate provision for the special requirements for the study and treatment of the cases in each class, and the hospital must not be so crowded as to prevent adequate classification and treatment.

11. The classification must include a separate reception and intensive study and treatment department or building, a special

* American Journal of Psychiatry, Vol. 5, No. 2, October, 1925, p. 303.

unit for acute physical illnesses and surgical conditions, and separate units for the tuberculous, and the infirm and bedfast. Each of these units must be suitably organized and equipped for the requirements of the class of patients under treatment.

12. The hospital must be provided with a clinical and pathological laboratory, equipped and manned in accordance with the minimum standards recommended by the Committee on Pathological Investigation.

13. The hospital must be provided with adequate X-ray equipment and employ a well qualified radiologist.

14. There must be a working medical library and journal file.

15. The treatment facilities and equipment must include:

(a) A fully equipped surgical operating room.

(b) A dental office supplied with modern dental equipment.

(c) Tubs and other essential equipment for hydrotherapy operated by one or more specially trained physiotherapists.

(d) Adequately equipped examination rooms for the specialties in medicine and surgery required by the schedule.

(e) Provision for occupational therapy and the employment of specially trained instructors.

(f) Provision for treatment by physical exercises and games and the employment of specially trained instructors.

(g) Adequate provision for recreation and social entertainment.

16. Regular staff conferences must be held at least twice a week where the work of the physicians and the examination and treatment of the patients will be carefully reviewed. Minutes of the conference must be kept.

17. There must be one or more out-patient clinics conducted by the hospital in addition to any on the hospital premises. An adequate force of trained social workers must be employed.

18. There must be an adequate nursing force, in the proportion to total patients of not less than 1 to 8, and to the patients of intensive treatment and acute sick and surgical units of not less than 1 to 4. Provision must be made for adequate systematic instruction and training of the members of the nursing force.

19. Mechanical restraint and seclusion, if used at all, must be under strict regulations and a system of control and record by the physicians, and must be limited to the most urgent conditions."

Surely the state hospital that measures up to these requirements has come a long way from the old asylum of the nineteenth century.

Scientific progress takes place in accordance with certain laws and is stimulated by certain events. The fabrication of a new instrument like the microscope, the invention of a new method like the staining of tissues, are tremendously important and significant events for scientific progress. New instruments and new methods are at once appropriated and applied to the solution of problems in all directions so far as possible. Improvements of the instrument are brought about, as are elaborations and refinements of the method, and progress continues along these lines until a time comes when the limits of instrument and method have been practically reached and when further expectations from these sources can only be additional facts discovered along the same lines, nothing essentially new. The instrument and the method have been exhausted, at least for the time being.

Now there is another stimulus for scientific research that is equally as important as new instruments and new methods, and that is new ideas, new points of view, new ways of looking at facts, new concepts, a new order of values, in fact an entirely different orientation toward the whole subject matter under investigation; such a new orientation, for example, as came from the study of astronomy, from considering the earth as the center of the universe and therefore the most important and most significant of all heavenly bodies, made purposely as a habitation for man, designed for his convenience and happiness. The geocentric theory of the universe forever confined scientific thought and progress within a very narrow horizon. This horizon was broken through and enlarged when the falsity of this position was discovered and the geocentric theory was discarded and the real place of the earth in the cosmos began to be appreciated. The same comments might be made with reference to man's place in nature before the development of the evolution hypothesis, and the result of discarding the immature ideas of this pre-evolutionary period and accepting the wider and more significant views that came with the advent of evolution and the understanding of man's relationship to the whole of organic nature.

A similar change took place in the evaluation of man's mind and in the understanding of its significance and the appreciation of its structure and functions when psychoanalysis made its appearance. This happened in the early years of the century. As a matter of fact, I had run across Breuer and Freud's book, " Über Hysterie," back in the early days when I was working with Sidis at the Pathological Institute on Madison Avenue, but Sidis had not thought much of the book, apparently, and so I did not pay much attention to it. But in the next few years we began to hear the reverberations of this movement as they came across from Vienna; and in this country the cause of psychoanalysis was early espoused by Dr. Ernest Jones, who first lived in Canada—Toronto, I think, and subsequently came to the United States, and by Dr. A. A. Brill, of New York, who became the translator of Professor Sigmund Freud's works. The first record I have of the organization of any psychoanalytic societies in this country was in 1910; and three years later, in 1913, Dr. Jelliffe and I, after a great deal of preliminary consultation with various people—historians, anthropologists, psychologists, etc.— launched *The Psychoanalytic Review*. At about the same time the movement had received sufficient emphasis to have created a considerable amount of antagonism. Dr. Brill and Dr. Jones and a small group of us had been pretty continuously at work. I had published my book on Mental Mechanisms (1911). The International Course in Neurology and Psychiatry had been given at Fordham University in 1912, where I had lectured and to which Dr. Jung was invited to give a course of lectures. So that the movement was gaining, in definition at least, if only slightly in proportions. The antagonisms came along swiftly, however, with the progress of the movement, and seemed pretty generally to be related to the emphasis that the movement placed upon the sex instinct. This can easily be understood because of the absolute blindness of the nineteenth century in this respect. The nineteenth century believed in ignorance and silence. Psychoanalysis believed in neither and the result was, probably largely because of the enthusiasms of its proponents, that sex instead of having its rightful place of importance was probably overemphasized, for, as Professor William James used to say, we can not have anything in this world without having too much of it. The antagonism took many forms, but I remember very well one of the leading professors of neurology in this country saying to me at Fordham University during the course in the Fall of 1912—or at least putting his comment in the form of a question by asking me whether I did not believe that the psychoanalytic movement had run its course and was then diminishing. The course of events subsequently obviously demonstrates this to have been a bit of wishful thinking.

The thing that psychoanalysis did for psychiatry was to open a door to the understanding of the patient which strangely had always heretofore been closed; and one reason that it had always been closed was that the physician had never paid very much, if any, attention to what the patient said, putting his remarks down as of no significance because they were crazy or incoherent. Much less did the physician in the old days ever have the slightest idea that these crazy, incoherent remarks might by any chance have a meaning. Psychoanalysis oriented the physician toward his patient in an entirely different way. It promulgated the doctrine of psychic determinism. It considered the patient as an organism and expected to find causes of psychic events, just as surely as it might be expected to find causes of psychical events, and therefore for the psychoanalyst everything the patient said necessarily had significance and in accordance with the postulates of science this significance could be found in the antecedents of his remarks. Causes precede effects, and effects somehow are potential in their causes. There was also the hypothesis of the unconscious, not so easy to understand but tremendously helpful when grasped, and which in a nutshell was, in substance, that the field of conscious awareness is not all there is to the mind.

I was ready for these psychoanalytic concepts because of the work that I had done with Sidis in studying the problems of mental dissociation and double personality. I was accustomed to sit by the patient's bedside with pencil and paper and take down religiously everything that he said, hoping to find among these broken fragments of his discourse some leading line that would be of significance and importance. I was accustomed to listening to these delirioid utterances and expecting to be able to hitch them up with actual occurrences in the life of the patient, and I even expected that this was, theoretically at least, possible to the minutest detail. I had perhaps never formulated definitely the theory of psychic determinism but I acted " as if " I had, and the concept was therefore not alien to my way of thinking and acting. I even remember that when I was studying one case the patient used a word which I could not understand and which sounded strange, perhaps as if it might be in a strange language. I insisted upon endeavoring to find out the significance of this word, and lo and behold, finally the significance emerged. The name was a word of a foreign language, but it was the name of a racehorse upon which my patient had bet his last penny and had won a small amount of money, with which money he had purchased some cigarettes. In his delirium he had designated these cigarettes by the name of the racehorse—obviously a confusing procedure on his part but my theory of the necessary significance of such apparently meaningless productions was justified. So when psychoanalysis came along offering the same sort of thing it was perfectly acceptable, to my way of thinking.

In 1914 the American Medico-Psychological Association had its

annual meeting in Baltimore. At that time the antagonism to psychoanalysis had become quite marked and its enemies desired to bring
the matter to a head and to quash it for all time. The President of
the Association, a man for whom I had the greatest respect and who
was a man of great ability, in fact the man who as President of the
then so-called Lunacy Commission of New York State had adminis-
tratively organized New York State's hospital system, was Dr. Carlos
F. MacDonald. He was well known to be violently opposed to the
psychoanalytic movement. On the program a paper was presented
which tore the whole movement to shreds. This paper was by my
friend, Dr. Charles W. Burr, of Philadelphia. Following this paper
there was an elaborate discussion, carefully prepared and reduced to
writing, by Dr. F. X. Dercum, also of Philadelphia. Following these
broadsides against the psychoanalytic movement I arose to speak on
the other side of the case and, I believe, made my first public defense
of psychoanalysis. In turning to the Transactions of the Association
for that year I find my remarks reported as follows:*

> " Of course it is entirely impossible to deal with these two
> papers in the few minutes at my disposal, but I think something
> should be said, even though I feel that I have been pretty well
> raked over the coals by the speakers, because I am in sympathy
> with psychoanalysis. Psychoanalysis, speaking very simply, pre-
> tends to do with the human mind what we learned to do with the
> human body hundreds of years ago; we had to learn to dissect the
> human body to find out what it was made of, just in the same
> way they have got to learn to dissect the human mind to find out
> what it is made of, and our efforts to do that dissection of the
> human mind must be made in the face of just about the same kind
> of arguments, the same kind of prejudices that hampered the
> efforts to dissect the human body years and years ago; every
> scientific advance, every step forward, every opening of a new
> door is made the same source of the same kind of resistances. I
> am entirely in harmony with Dr. Burr when he says that it does
> not make any difference about the type of the individual who
> stands for a certain doctrine; I have no feeling against the people
> who make this resistance; I consider them of value in the com-
> munity. Galileo said he saw satellites about Jupiter and people
> said there was no such thing; there was nothing like that in the
> Bible. He said he had a telescope through which you could look
> and see these satellites; they said it was a sin to look through a
> telescope, and even if you did look through it the telescope was
> made with the satellites in it.

* Discussion of "A Criticism of Psychoanalysis" by Dr. Charles W. Burr.
Proceedings Amer. Medico-Psychological Ass'n, Vol. 21, 1914, p. 322.

" Dr. Burr has presented certain cases, certain clinical records and dismissed the subject by saying the whole thing was absurd; he did not bring forth any specific argument. A society of this sort should be the proper arena where such things should be threshed out on scientific merits; prejudices should not enter into the question at all. I am a psychoanalyst; I want the truth and I am willing to welcome any light that may be thrown upon the situation. I appreciate psychoanalysis for I have been confused by actual clinical contact with patients in regard to the underlying principles and meanings involved and so I know there is an element of truth in the whole movement, which would be extremely unfortunate for us to discard at this point. It is not the criticism of psychoanalysis that has been presented; I have no doubt that many hypotheses will be laughed at in years to come as being in fault, perhaps some of them ridiculous, but what we want is their correction at this point; we want more light; we want more truth; it does not do any good to call them absurd and let the matter go at that. Why not when dealing with psychological things stick to them; why must people go back of them to physical things until we are ready; while we are on the road let us deal frankly with the psychological subjects and not presume anything we do not know. Now, I anticipate for psychoanalysis an attitude of open-mindedness toward a movement which is endeavoring to help a certain type of sick individuals. It is not true that the psychoanalyst always seeks for certain repressed sexual features. The psychoanalyst deals with the patient in a difficulty; he tries to find out what the difficulty is and how to help the patient out of the difficulty, just as every other physician does, and he does not jump at a whole lot of make-believe things. It may be true of certain beginners who do not understand it. We have to follow the patient and never lead him. We do not know when a dream is told to us what the translation means; we have no possible way of knowing. When the psychanalyst speaks himself of being cocksure, when he speaks with certain assurance before the other physician who does not understand such things, he is suffering from something which cannot be laid at the door of psychanalysis. Psychanalysis is a method and as a result of the method certain things have been uncovered, which are facts, whether they exist in the mind of the patient, the psychanalyst, or anywhere else, and those facts must receive some interpretation; if our interpretation is wrong, there is a right interpretation, and I ask the people who criticize the movement to come forward and tell us what all these things mean. We offer our explanation; we are willing to withdraw if we are wrong.

" I trust this society will maintain an open attitude toward this subject. I will only say one word more: I think very largely the difficulty of understanding the whole psychoanalytical movement is a lack of understanding of what is meant by the unconscious; that is an extremely difficult concept to get. I have spent many months in getting a clear idea about it, and I would invite your attention especially to that feature. It is not strange that the psychanalyst should say that he has thrown a certain light on these things. We have, many years, been studying the human mind; we have gone deeper and deeper into the explanation of mental actions, and welcome any light that can be thrown on the human mind.

"What I have said is a simple statement of fact. Now I believe there are others who also want to speak a few moments and so I will stop."

I should perhaps have liked to have smoothed out certain rough spots in the English, but in the main these remarks represented my position at that time and I therefore reproduce them here.

From this time on the psychoanalytic movement progressed, slowly gaining additional adherents but, perhaps rather unfortunately, gaining popular support much more rapidly so that the general body of information might be said to have been pretty superficial and for the most part erroneous. The public were intrigued but not well informed. It is not my purpose to trace in detail the history of what happened during the years, except to recall progress and to indicate in what it consisted in the most obvious instances. The little body of original workers increased in size. Brill and Jelliffe continued to render yeoman's service to the movement. The publication of Dr. Edward J. Kempf's large work on Psychopathology was a notable addition to the American literature, while the translations of Freud and other European analysts had begun to appear. There were, of course, many other contributors to the movement, some of them notable, but the main point is that the movement grew and in spite of all the predictions to the contrary has become firmly established.

Perhaps in some respects the most important thing that psychoanalysis did for psychiatry, and for that matter for medicine at large, was, as I have already indicated, to show the value of listening to what the patient had to say, or, as I like to call it, the language of disease. The language of disease, of course, is not always a spoken language. The heart murmur or the pulmonary râle or the pulse beat, the thermometer, the metabolism apparatus,—all speak the language of disease. The general practitioner was familiar with these particular dialects, but as to the spoken language that is formulated in words and with which the patient undertakes to communicate his thoughts and feelings or to express himself,—this language had been sadly neglected. It might, too, be commented upon that heretofore anybody felt himself to be competent to pass upon another's state of mind, and this is true even now very largely. The layman, the lawyer, or the legislator, who would not think of differing from the opinion of his physician when he is told what was found as a result of a urine examination or a cystoscopy, or what not, will glibly express himself regarding the sanity or otherwise of an individual after perhaps only a few casual questions. The idea seems to be pretty firmly fixed that a knowledge of psychology is the gift of everyone, that in correspondence with his experience with others this knowledge, to be sure, may be enlarged, but after all anybody can tell whether another person is crazy, or reasonable, or what not; all of which implies that there are no particular laws that govern the operation of the mind, that there is no particular technique for discovering what is going on in the mind, that everyone interprets what he hears and sees from his own point of view. Psychoanalysis did very much to modify this exceedingly naïve assumption and demonstrated that mental events, like physical events, are not always what they seem, that the patient is not always testifying to the facts when he tells you what he thinks and feels, even though he may firmly believe that he is, that there are laws that govern the operation of the mind, that there are techniques and methods for discovering what is going on in the mind of the patient. Psychoanalysis not only helped to bring about this changed attitude toward psychic events, but it also demonstrated that what the patient says and what actually goes on in the mind are important, that they are not just casual things that pass by, that they have significance—sometimes very great significance, and that many of the mental symptoms which have been passed over heretofore as just being evidences of delirium, or distraction, or what not, really are important to understand if one is to understand one's patient.

Dr. Jelliffe and I from the very first were convinced of the importance of the psychoanalytic attack upon and knowledge of the individual; and we were convinced of its importance for general medicine and we have never lost an opportunity to emphasize this. Others, to be sure, have done the same thing; but it is exceedingly satisfactory after all these years to find that general medicine is, as a matter of fact, beginning to recognize the psychological point of view, although in many instances, of course, it has not the remotest idea of the connection of this point of view with the story of psychoanalysis.

So as compared with what happened in Baltimore in 1914 what a different picture is presented in 1927, when on the occasion of the seventy-eighth annual session of the American Medical Association, in Washington, the section on the Practice of Medicine held a symposium on Psychic and Emotional Factors in Disease. In this symposium there were several papers, read by the cardiologist, the gastro-enterologist, and others; and, as the matter lies roughly in my memory, the testimony of all these specialists was to the effect that approximately 50 per cent of the patients who came to their offices presented no physical findings, that is, there was nothing organic wrong with them that was discoverable. At the close of this symposium I responded to an invitation to make a few remarks; and to indicate concretely what had happened in the intervening thirteen years, and my state of mind upon this particular occasion, I will introduce these remarks in full, as follows:

" Mr. Chairman, Ladies and Gentlemen: I am very glad to respond to this invitation. Let me tell you why. I made a considerable effort to get here this morning, very frankly, not especially to hear what the readers of papers had to say in their various papers (although I have been deeply interested in what they did say, and I am glad to express my appreciation of what I consider to be very valuable contributions on the part of the readers), but I came here because I believed this was really a historical occasion. Some few of us in the realm of psychopathology have always had a great faith that ultimately the psyche or the mind of the patient would come in for proper recognition in the general practice of medicine. Why it has not in the past is perhaps a long story. I have my own feeling about it. I have a suspicion that the conservative factor in medicine has operated in conjunction with the early teachings of the church that have allied for two thousand years the flesh and the devil, so that we have always been anxious to hitch upon the body all of the sins of the soul. If we can project upon a certain organ of the body some of our sinfulness, we, I am sure, will not find any serious difficulty in getting a surgeon to cut it out. Then everybody ought to be satisfied.

"As I said, I believe this is a historical occasion. As I very often say, the mind didn't come into the picture of evolution at some particular point, didn't attach itself to the body in an extraneous sort of way—the way a crow perches itself upon a telegraph pole. The psychic factors of the organism are as much a part of it as the somatic factors and if we were to consider the organism as a crystal, for example, the psychic components represent only one of its facets. And so we psychopathologists have always believed that the people who were really treating the psychoneuroses were all medical specialists except the psychiatrists.

"When I come into this meeting, devoted to a consideration of the psychic factors of somatic disease, and see a large room like this crowded to the walls, I naturally feel that a hope that I have entertained for years has come to fruition. It isn't that the physicians have not recognized psychic factors in the past. They have been recognized very definitely two thousand years ago, but it is one thing for the occasional physician to recognize them; it is one thing for them to be recognized intuitively and unconsciously; and it is an entirely different thing for that recognition to be made conscious and to become the possession of the entire profession. I feel that this meeting symbolizes the beginning of that self-consciousness on the part of the medical profession of the importance of the psychic factors in disease and I feel that it is a great privilege to have had the opportunity to say just these few words to you upon this occasion, and I feel in closing that we should all congratulate ourselves for being here and I trust that the future will prove that my hopes and aspirations for the recognition of the mind in medicine will be demonstrated to have had really initial impetus at this meeting this morning."

It will be seen from the title of this symposium that general medicine, so far as it had gone along in accepting the importance of the psychological aspects of disease, had also incidentally accepted another tenet of the psychoanalyst, probably again without realizing its source, and that tenet is that mental disorder by and large is a matter of the emotions and not of the intelligence. A man may be able to answer all the ordinary questions that tax his memory and his intelligence and yet be exceedingly and seriously ill mentally. This is indeed promising and even though some of the pioneers who are responsible for the beginning of this great new movement in medicine, as it seems to me to be, do not get personal credit for what has happened and for what they think is their due, nevertheless they have to be prepared to be sufficiently repaid by the results, and, like parents, be glad to see their children successful even though those same children have not the remotest idea how much they owe their parents and never will have until they in turn become parents.

From 1927 on the movement has continued to progress. Psychoanalysis, as everyone knows, has become a vast body of thought that branches out in all directions, not only in therapeutics but in psychology, anthropology, sociology, art, religion, and in fact in every direction in which man's interests lead him. It has been more and more accepted by medicine. It is beginning to be taught here and there in the departments of psychiatry in medical schools. The psychiatrist, particularly of the psychopathic hospitals and wards, is using it, sometimes perhaps without knowing it but nevertheless he is using it, often consciously; an increasing number of journals are being devoted to it; and institutes are springing up here and there where the young physician may qualify himself for its practice. The standards of these institutes are maintained upon an international basis and of the highest character, the desirable amount of time for completing a course being put at four years, during which the applicant is himself analyzed, completes at least two control analyses, and in the meantime attends numerous lectures and seminars where the experience of all of those connected with the institute is freely exchanged. In addition to this, hospitals for mental disease are beginning to have analysts on their staffs, in two instances at least permitting members of the staff extended leave of absence so that they may equip themselves in this field of therapy. So that progress in the therapeutics of mental disease is proceeding apace.

It must not be supposed, however, that with all this activity it has always been smooth sailing. The antagonism to the analytic movement continues to be marked and in spots violent. Occasional blunders, particularly in the early days, which led to tragic results, of course did not help matters; and even now from time to time cases come to attention which have gotten worse under analysis, and once in a while a patient commits suicide. When these things happen they are all used as arguments against analysis; and yet it seems to me that what they really indicate is that analysis is a major operation, and like all major procedures where life and death are involved, as they frequently are in these malignant psychotic conditions—if not the bodily life, then the mental, which is equally or more important— success does not always crown our efforts. The surgeon does not always save his patient's life, neither will the analyst; but experience is getting richer every day and we are learning more and more how to deal with these difficult problems.

In addition to all these things that have happened, the recent years since the War have shown a reversal of the flow of visitors. In the pre-war period doctors always went to Europe. In the post-war period the doctor frequently comes to America from Europe. During these years we have seen a number of the leading analysts and psychiatrists of Europe. Freud came here, along with Jung, in the early days, to lecture at Worcester; and in recent years Dr. Sándor Ferenczi and Dr. Wilhelm Stekel and Dr. Otto Rank and Dr. Paul Federn have been here, while at the present moment Dr. Franz Alexander is in Boston, Dr. H. Nunberg is in Philadelphia, Dr. Sándor

Radó and Dr. Paul Schilder are in New York—to say nothing of quite a group of physicians in New York City who have been analyzed by Freud, and a scattering of others throughout the country who have returned from Europe after having studied with one or another of the more prominent European analysts. And so the matter stands. A great advance has been made from the psychological side of medicine. It was initiated by psychoanalysis. Psychoanalysis has advanced during the years very considerably and yet there is still a very pronounced, a very definite, and a very strong movement against it.

As an indication of my feeling toward the whole psychoanalytic movement as it existed in 1914—and for that matter as it still exists, I find the following letter in my files:

" Washington, D. C., October 20th, 1914

" Karolinska Institutet,
   Den Medicinska Nobelkomiten,
     Stockholm, Sweden.

" Gentlemen:

" I have the honor to acknowledge your communication, dated September 1914, inviting me to propose a candidate for the Nobel Prize in the section Physiology and Medicine, which is intended for distribution during the year 1915.

" I have the honor to propose the name of Professor Sigmund Freud, of Vienna.

" My motives for proposing the name of Professor Freud are that in my opinion his work has opened a new era in mental medicine. By his study of the psychology of neurotics he has been enabled to interpret mental symptoms, which before were meaningless. In fact, the whole field of psychopathology is indebted to his methods of interpretation, and whatever difference of opinion may exist as to a particular interpretation in a particular instance or the specific meaning attributable to a certain symptom, the method of approach to these psychological problems by psychoanalysis is a distinct methodological contribution to medicine of undoubtedly enormous value.

" Professor Freud's writings are numerous, the most important of which are ' Traumdeutung,' ' Psychopathologie des Alltagslebens,' and his ' Neurosenlehre.' Besides these works there are a great number of contributions to the journal literature, of which perhaps the most important are ' Psychoanalytische Bemerkungen über einen autobiographisch beschriebenen Fall von Paranoia (Dementia paranoides),' and ' Totem und Tabu,' published in Imago.

        " Very respectfully,
           "(Signed)   Wm. A. White."

## CHAPTER X

THE HYGIENE OF THE MIND—PREVENTION—A POSITIVE HEALTH
PROGRAM

As I have already indicated several times, it is impossible to tell this story of psychiatry in two dimensions. Of the many things that happened during the forty-year period many of them happened at approximately the same time and a great many of them had their inception at the beginning of the century. It was at the beginning of the century that the psychoanalytic movement began to show itself, and it was at the beginning of the century that the mental hygiene movement also began to take on form. These two movements since that time have been running parallel but by no means unrelated to each other. In fact it would be a little difficult to see how the hygiene of the mind could have been developed in the old days when psychiatry was purely a descriptive matter and its patients were all in asylums. Even the illumination of Kraepelin's great work could hardly have had as one of its results a mental hygiene movement that would have had any vitality, because after all Kraepelin was still a descriptive psychiatrist. In order that the problem of mental hygiene should be tackled it was necessary that some meaning should be discovered in the symptoms of the psychoses, and it was by giving these symptoms a meaning that the psychoanalytic movement made its greatest contribution to mental hygiene.

The mental hygiene movement had its inception in the experiences of Mr. Clifford W. Beers. He had been a patient in several institutions for mental disease and found himself at the end of his experience so outraged by what he considered the stupid and cruel way in which he had been treated that he prepared the manuscript of his book " A Mind That Found Itself," and set about consulting various psychiatrists and public-minded men for the purpose of determining upon a plan whereby such conditions might be relieved. As a result of his activities the first Mental Hygiene Society was formed in the State of Connecticut on the 6th of May, 1908, while a few months later, namely, in February of the following year, the National Committee for Mental Hygiene was

brought into existence. Acknowledgment should be made to
Dr. Adolf Meyer for suggesting the very apt and appropriate term
" mental hygiene." No one, of course, can tell how much influence
the right name may have upon a movement such at this, but everyone will concede that to all appearances it has been a most happy
one. Naturally, from the way in which it originated the mental
hygiene movement had as its first objective the improvement in the
treatment of the so-called " insane " in our great public institutions,
principally the state hospitals, and this improvement looked primarily to the development of greater intelligence on the part of the
care-takers, to the elimination of cruelty and the abuses of restraint
and isolation, and in general, therefore, to a realization in practice
of that humanitarian attitude which was symbolized by Pinel's
liberation of the " insane " at the Salpêtrière. Twenty-two years
later, in my Presidential Address to the First International Congress
on Mental Hygiene * I described the origin of the mental hygiene
movement in the following way:

" The way in which the mental hygiene movement originally
came into being seems to me of the utmost significance. It was
not the outgrowth of any philosophy started by a group who
were bound to prove that the tenets of that philosophy were
sound. It was infinitely more simple. Its objective—and its
sole objective except for some broader formulations regarding
prevention and research that appeared even in its first statements—was in its earliest days the improvement of the care
of the so-called ' insane.' Mr. Beers was convinced by personal
experience that this care was not what it should be, that its
defects were due to ignorance largely, to lack of understanding
of the mental patient and of proper standards of care in institutions, and he set about in a constructive way to correct the
evils as he saw them. As you see, a perfectly simple procedure.
Certain things were wrong. What could be done to improve
them? Here was a program with which no one could find fault.
As soon as presented, it necessarily found agreement on all
hands. And so the movement was launched in this way. The
attitude of mind that animated those who were originally involved
was one with which we are perfectly familiar. It has been the
attitude through the ages of the physician. He sees things
that produce unhappiness and suffering and he tries to correct
them. He does not wait until all of the scientific and philosophical questions that could be raised surrounding the particular

* White, W. A.: The Origin, Growth and Significance of the Mental
Hygiene Movement. Mental Hygiene, Vol. 14, No. 3, July, 1930, p. 555;
Science, Vol. 72, No. 1856, July 25, 1930, p. 77.

situation are solved, nor does he alter his treatment according to whether he considers his various types of patient more or less worth while.   Mental hygiene did not stop to solve the metaphysical, philosophical and theological problems that have always been associated with the study of the mind.   It did not seriously consider such questions as the freedom of the will or the relation of body and mind or the moral factors that were involved in mental illness, but accepted man just as it found him, with his hates and loves, his hopes, fears, wishes, aspirations and ideals, and tried to find a better solution for his difficulties than he had been able to.   It is precisely the attitude of the surgeon at the operating table to whom is brought a man with a bullet wound.   He does not stop to inquire how the wound was received, whether in the commission of a crime or in the defense of his home, but proceeds at once to see how matters can be made better.   He feels it to be his duty to give the best he has of his skill then and there to that particular patient without qualification.   That is what the practice of medicine means to him and has meant down the ages.   Back of this way of going at things lies the tacit assumption that human life is in itself valuable, that it is worth while to save it and that the way in which it is lived can often be improved with a little help."

It was natural after the mental hygiene movement got under way that it should develop in the first place a systematic procedure; and one of the main features of this systematic procedure was to make a survey of the different states of the Union at the invitation of the authorities of these states and to make a report with recommendations looking toward the improvement of the care of the "insane" in the state, these improvements comprising recommendations along the line of legislation, construction, and administration.   To date practically every state in the Union has been so surveyed.   Many of the improvements in the condition of the "insane" are traceable to the results of these surveys.

Naturally, too, after the ground had been well broken in this work of improving the condition of the "insane," the National Committee turned to the improvement of the condition of the defective, also confined in great state institutions.   In this work it was largely guided by the judgment of the late Dr. Walter E. Fernald, then Superintendent of the State Institution for the Feebleminded at Waverley, Massachusetts, and who has been called the Father of the Feebleminded in this country.   His wise judgment guided the Committee in this new territory to good effect and ever since they have kept up their interest in this aspect of the work.

Following this it was but natural that the most neglected of all persons cared for by the state, the criminal, should receive similar consideration.  The National Committee had interested itself in the criminal but not quite so extensively as in the " insane " and the feebleminded.  But this work in prisons is recognized as a very important one and dates its inception from the work of Dr. Bernard Glueck, for some years in charge of the prison department of Saint Elizabeths Hospital and drafted into the mental hygiene movement by Dr. Thomas W. Salmon, then Medical Director of the National Committee for Mental Hygiene, who induced him to make a study of the admissions to Sing Sing Prison (1916–1917).*  The result of this work had a profound influence upon the attitude toward the prisoner, and from that time until the present there has been a steady tendency for the psychiatrist and the psychologist to find a niche for himself in the prison system.

These were the activities that interested the National Committee for Mental Hygiene during the early years of its existence.  In turning to their Hand Book of the Mental Hygiene Movement, which they published in 1913, I find among other things the following statements: There were on January 1, 1910, 187,454 " insane " in the institutions of the United States.  This figure was compared with the total number of officers and enlisted men in the United States Army, Navy and Marine Corps, 142,695; the total number of students in colleges and universities in the United States, 184,712; the population of Columbus, Ohio, the twenty-ninth largest city in the United States, 181,548.  The annual cost of these 187,454 patients, calculated on the basis of $175 per capita, was $32,804,450.  This was compared with the cost of completing the Panama Canal, which was $325,201,000, as approximately one-tenth of that amount, namely, $32,520,100; and the cost of this Canal was so great that is was paid for over a period of ten years, 1904 to 1914.  The cost of caring for the " insane " in one of the States, which I believe must have been New York State, is one of the largest elements in the budget, the largest portion of the budget, namely, 24 per cent, being devoted to education, the next largest,

* Glueck, Bernard:  A Study of 608 Admissions to Sing Sing Prison. Mental Hygiene, Vol. 2, No. 1, Jan., 1918, p. 85.

namely, 23 per cent, being devoted to the care of the "insane."
There are a number of other exceedingly interesting statements,
one of which we shall perhaps refer to again, and that is that the
deaths from smallpox in the entire United States in 1911 were
134, whereas the deaths from general paresis during the same period
in New York State alone were 590.  The Hand Book is further
illustrated by pictures of restraint apparatus as compared with
the continuous bath now used; the hopeless, idle, miserable surroundings of the "insane" in county almshouses as compared
with the industrious group in the pleasant surroundings provided
by the modern state hospital.

As compared with the above statistics, the statistics as we have
them today are significant.  If the statisticians tell us correctly,
there are now walking the streets of the United States one million
young people who will spend some portion of their time before
they die in an institution for mental diseases.  There are today
throughout the United States in all the hospitals of all kinds and
descriptions approximately 800,000 beds, of which approximately
one-half, or 400,000, are for mental patients.  A recent survey of
the situation in New York State indicated that one resident of
New York State in every twenty-five would at some time during
his life find his way into an institution for mental disease.  Whereas
the statisticians calculate that in 1970 these United States will have
attained to a stable population, assuming that things will go on as
they have in the past, of 150,000,000 of people, and of this number
950,000 will be in institutions for mental disease, or more than
double the number at present so cared for.  All these figures and
the tendencies shown by them have indicated very clearly that
mental disease is much more prevalent than was formerly supposed,
for it can hardly be true that these figures represent an increase
in this group of maladies.  Statistics for mental disease go back
only to 1880, and in that brief period the statistical increase has
been enormous.  It can not be true that conditions have so radically
changed as to account for this.  What is probably true is that mental
disease is being discovered.  The public institutions are gaining the
confidence of the people and they are being sought where before
they were avoided.  The concept of mental disease has been
liberalized so that many conditions which would not have been
included in the past are now included.  These are the more probable

reasons for this rather alarming statistical showing. Be that as it may, the indications are clear that we are not handling the problem by any means in an effective way. The National Committee, therefore, came to feel rather early in the story, really, that mental disease was in the very largest sense of the term a public health problem and as such the most potent way to attack this problem was by means of the application of preventive principles. So the term " mental hygiene " comes into its true significance when it is coupled with a program of prevention.

In examining this question of the statistics of mental disease I took occasion to study the mortality statistics as recorded in the United States Census reports. The net result of this study was that it was shown that the death ratio in the general population was 13.1 per thousand, while the death ratio in institutions for mental disease was 74.3. So that in spite of the fact that the institution for mental disease is built in order to provide an environment which removes the stress from its patient population, nevertheless Dame Nature takes her toll by way of the differential death rate. Whatever may be the developments of the preventive program and whatever may be the practical changes that are made in handling this great mass of relatively inadequate personalities, there issues from this survey the conviction that mental health is not just the result of preventing mental disease but that it represents a positive goal to be striven for. With reference to this particular aspect of the movement, I said in my Presidential Address previously quoted:

"I believe that the most significant change that mental hygiene is going to effect in the future will be a change in our concept of values as applied to human beings. I have indicated that the highest ideals that medicine had reached in the last century were the prevention of disease and the avoidance of death. These ideals, when applied in the mental field, were expressed in the well-known dictum, 'A sound mind in a sound body.' If, however, as I believe, living in order to avoid dying presents very little that is either worth while or stimulating as an ideal, so the concept of the sound mind in the sound body falls equally short of the truth, and in the same, namely, a negative, direction. The thought that I would like you to take away from the few words that I have said is that mental hygiene presents a positive program for life well lived, for mental health because of its values and not because of what it avoids. The value of life is measured by what we become, and so by the nature of the influences we radiate in our living. Life's values, from the standpoint of mental health, are not expressed in terms of the chemistry of nutrition or the integrity of the heart muscle or of any organ, but in terms of character, of man as a social being, of those effects which he produces on those about him, the enthusiasms he stimulates that go reverberating down the ages translated by the personalities that trace back to the original source. This is a tangible form of immortality toward which every one may strive with some show of success, and in the striving get out of life the most there is in it for him."

The ability to bring to pass a program of this tremendous significance will depend upon our knowledge of the mind and our ability to modify its reactions, particularly at the critical periods in life. Some overenthusiastic psychoanalysts seem to think that the salvation of the world depends upon everyone being analyzed. If it does, then I am afraid the world is hopelessly lost, for I cannot vision the time when any such possibility will be even remotely approximated. What we can do, however, is to strive to gather the information which the psychoanalysts and all the other students of the mind and of human behavior have to offer and try to fit it into a program that will make for mental health, which undoubtedly means modifications reaching all through our social system, particularly in the fields of education, religion, law, and medicine itself. The magnitude of such a program is appalling, but life-bearing systems have a way of surmounting difficulties and overcoming obstacles which when studied in the cold, logical formulae of the printed page appear to present impossibilities, and one whose eyes are as open for the facts of progress as for the signs of dissolution may look about him and see many indications that these modifications are already taking place.

The occurrence of the First International Congress on Mental Hygiene in 1930, with its representatives from every continent on the globe and upwards of fifty countries, with its membership of some four thousand and its attendance of three thousand, and the fact that during this Congress there was organized an International Committee for Mental Hygiene and that this Committee is now at work on the program for a Second International Congress on Mental Hygiene, intended to be held in Paris in 1935, give some indication of the extent to which interest in mental health has grown. In this country alone mental hygiene clinics have been springing up in every direction, so that the prospects are that there will be some approximation of ability to meet the needs in the course of a reasonable time. Further than this, more and more physicians are specializing in the psychiatric field; and at the present moment a special committee of the National Committee for Mental Hygiene has just made its report on medical education throughout the United States with reference to the teaching of psychiatry, which report constitutes the first step in stimulating the enlargement of the medical curricula so that students who graduate in medicine hereafter will have some training in psychiatry comparable to that which they get in other fields of medicine and which approximates the need as represented by the statistics which I have submitted.

# CHAPTER XI

## The Law and the Social Sciences

As I am in the habit of saying, the so-called " insane " have been pursued through the ages by three Furies—Ignorance, Superstition, and Fear. Each of these has in its own way added to the hardships which they have had to endure, and probably in no field of human endeavor is this seen more clearly than in the field covered by the law. Both legislation and legal practice have discriminated in an almost unbelievable way against the mentally ill. The trial of patients on the charge of " insanity " in order to commit them to insane asylums in its very statement gives an idea of the hopelessly inadequate conception of our legislatures and our legal profession regarding the various conditions of mental disease. And when in addition to this we find in certain jurisdictions as a pre-condition even to this unnecessary and humiliating procedure, a statement to the effect that the individual in order to be treated must, in the first place, be a pauper, although there is no other place than the public institution for a person with money to get treated in most jurisdictions, and, in the second place, must be dangerous,—we get some faint idea of the tremendous space that separates the thinking of the psychiatrist, who deals with the mental patient as a sick individual with the sole idea of restoring him to health, and the concept of the legal fraternity and the legislators, who see in him only a menace to their safety and take the necessary steps to secure his segregation. Nevertheless, in spite of this, progress does take place, although it comes to pass slowly and laboriously. At the present time I believe there are only seven States in the Union where the jury trial for the purposes of commitment has not been abandoned; but even in the jurisdictions where it has been abandoned for the most part at least, while the form has been changed the same primitive concepts rule and the proceeding as a whole has often not been greatly improved.

In 1824 a Royal Commission on Lunacy and Mental Disorder was appointed—

"(1) To inquire as regards England and Wales into the existing law and administrative machinery in connection with the certification, detention, and care of persons who are or are alleged to be of unsound mind.

"(2) To consider as regards England and Wales the extent to which provision is or should be made for the treatment without certification of persons suffering from mental disorder.

"And to make recommendations."

This commission made its report in 1926.* It was composed of a distinguished membership, largely of men learned in the law. The document is a voluminous one but a few excerpts from it may profitably be made as illustrating the tendency in modern lunacy legislation:

" The modern conception calls for the eradication of old-established prejudices and a complete revision of the attitude of society in the matter of its duty to the mentally afflicted " (p. 16).

" The keynote of the past has been detention; the keynote of the future should be prevention and treatment " (p. 17).

" Contrary to the accepted canons of preventive medicine, the mental patient is not admissible to most of the institutions provided for his treatment until his disease has progressed so far that he has become a certifiable lunatic. Then and then only is he eligible for treatment. It is, perhaps, not remarkable in these circumstances that the percentage of recoveries in public mental hospitals is low. In our view the position should be precisely reversed. Certification should be the last resort in treatment, not the prerequisite of treatment " (pp. 18–19).

" It is remarkable that in the case of a form of disease probably more subtle and difficult of diagnosis than any other, the layman should insist on his right to sit in judgment on the expert " (p. 20).

" If the true conception of a mental patient is that he is suffering from an illness, we can not help feeling that those who desire the further elaboration of legal machinery are apt to lose sight of the common sense of the matter " (p. 20).

" The problem of insanity is essentially a public health problem to be dealt with on modern public health lines. So only will the atmosphere of suspicion and aversion with which the subject is invested be dissipated " (p. 22).

In commenting upon the report of the Royal Commission a London correspondent said:

" Every facility should be afforded to the mentally ailing to submit voluntarily to treatment; but when compulsory detention is unavoidable, the intervention of the law should be as unobtrusive as possible."

These very admirable expressions indicate both what we are aiming at and how far we have fallen short of our goal.

* Report of the Royal Commission on Lunacy and Mental Disorder. Published by His Majesty's Stationery Office, London, 1926.

In the District of Columbia I have recommended a change in these archaic methods, and, in conjunction with various government and local agencies, I have succeeded in drafting a bill that contains the following provisions, which constitute the main changes from existing legislation:

(1) Provision for voluntary commitment for treatment, on request of patients, with provision for discharge on three days' notice.

(2) Provision that " insane " taken into custody by the police or other officials shall not be subjected to trials as are criminals, but may be held in the hospital and treated, and not tried except upon their requests or that of their relatives, guardians, or friends.

(3) If a trial is demanded by an " insane " person, his guardian, or friends, or by the court, upon petition, the "insane" person shall be heard by the court, and not subjected to trial by jury unless the " insane " person, his relatives, guardian, or friends demand it.

(4) Temporary commitment or detention is provided for, with provision that during such temporary commitment, and prior to formal commitment, the person may be released upon certificate to the District of Columbia by the superintendent of the hospital or by two physicians in regular attendance at any other hospital, that the person is not " insane " or has recovered his or her reason.

(5) Provision for the automatic restoration of the civil rights of patients discharged from the hospital on certificate of the superintendent that they are cured or that further treatment is unnecessary or undesirable.

The proposed legislation recommended, it is believed, would make unnecessary so many writs of habeas corpus, and would make simpler the release of patients to those competent to care for them. Up to the present writing, however, very little has been accomplished that would lead one to suppose that this bill is apt to become a law in the near future. Such is the extent of the cultural lag where the Three Furies are concerned.

Nevertheless, in spite of these disappointing circumstances, it is necessary in fairness to the facts to still say that progress is taking place. Year after year a more informed judiciary comes to handle these problems, and it comes with a mind into which something of the general attitude toward the " insane," which is slowly changing, has seeped, and we find the judges taking a more intelligent interest in the procession of patients that passes before them. The same improvement may be seen in whichever direction we look. For example, twenty-five years ago it was not uncommon for visitors to come to the hospital and ask to be shown the patients who were "chained" and were "in underground dungeons," and such like. Today visitors with such grotesque and morbid desires are very much rarer, or at least if they have such desires they do not express them. On the contrary, there is a marked increase in the number of visitors who come with a legitimate desire to know something about the institution, while with increasing frequency students from the nearby universities, colleges, and schools of one sort and another come in groups with their instructors to see certain aspects of the hospital,— students in sociology, students of abnormal psychology, parent-teachers associations who are becoming interested from another angle in their children, children who come to see how the dairy is run, visiting dietitians from other hospitals, etc., etc. So that despite the fact that the law sticks to its forms and to its methods of procedure it is being bombarded more and more forcibly each year and is yielding a little here and a little there, for it is fighting a losing fight against progress.

The same sort of criticisms might be leveled at the criminal law. For example, in my address before the joint session of the Section of Criminal Law and Criminology and the Judicial Section of the American Bar Association in 1927 * I said of the psychiatrist that:

> "He has come to feel that the criminal law and methods of legal procedure are based upon concepts which are largely obsolete from his point of view, and that penal methods as they at present exist are quite inadequate to deal with problems of human behavior."

The law has, through the ages, been interested almost solely in the forbidden act whereas the psychiatrist has equally been almost exclusively interested in the person who commits the forbidden act, the actor; and from these two standpoints there has been very little mutual understanding and very little possibility of a meeting of minds. The law, because of its lack of information about human beings, has relied almost solely upon punishment and fear to prevent certain acts. The psychiatrist, who knows much more about human beings, realizes that neither of these appeals is very effective, that in fact both of them not infrequently produce the results that they are calculated to prevent, and so naturally psychiatry can have very little sympathy with legalistic methods.

* White, W. A.: The Need for Coöperation between the Legal Profession and the Psychiatrist in Dealing with the Crime Problem. Amer. Journal of Psychiatry, Vol. 7, No. 3, Nov., 1927, p. 493.

It is always, of course, a rather easy thing for the minority to maintain a critical attitude toward those in power, and it is always easy to find fault and almost as easy to justify one's faultfinding if one is careful not to go to too great extremes. And so the psychiatrist has been pretty critical of the law and of legalistic methods, yet on the other hand I suspect that because of his lack of knowledge of these very highly specialized aspects of culture he would find himself in a rather difficult situation if he were suddenly asked, for example, to take over complete control of the administration of the prison system, all of which means that bad as law may be in its present archaic tendencies it has had a history which if we investigate it will disclose the fact that it developed methods along the way to suit conditions under restrictions and difficulties which made those methods often valuable at the time they came into being. The principal trouble now is that they continue to exist in a world that is radically different from the world in which they originated. In my address before mentioned I made the following concrete suggestions for improvement:

" 1. I believe fully in society's right to segregate the dangerous anti-social types so long as they continue dangerous. This means largely the doing away with fixed sentences, at least for certain types of crime, and making the return to freedom conditional upon some change in the individual that gives one a right to suppose that perhaps he will function more effectively as a social unit than he has in the past.

" 2. The elimination of punishment as a vengeance motive and its retention only if used for definitely constructive ends for conditioning conduct.

" 3. The gradual transformation of prisons into laboratories for the study of human behavior and the conditioning of human conduct.

" 4. The abolition in the trial of the hypothetical question.

" 5. The discarding of the concept of responsibility. The idea of responsibility is, as I have said, largely a metaphysical one. People who act anti-socially society must be protected from. So far as possible this should be done without raising metaphysical questions. How they should be cared for is a matter depending on what sort of persons they are and does not require a consideration of such abstruse matters.

" 6. The making of the positions of district attorney and of judges of criminal courts permanent positions and the appointment thereto a result of competitive examination protected by civil service laws. The requirements for filling such positions should be a knowledge of modern criminology in its various ramifications.

" 7. I think it would be an excellent thing, and I see no reason why it should not be done, to have such district attorneys and such judges in the course of their educational preparation serve internships in psychiatric clinics and prisons, just as physicians do in their various medical specialties."

Perhaps one of the most significant things that has happened in the whole legal territory has been the creation of the juvenile court, which came into existence in the first years of the century. Despite the fact that the method of procedure and the legislative enactments which brought these courts into existence in the several states are different in each instance, the fact remains that there has been set up a legal institution for dealing with certain types of individuals in the community who are not regarded, from the point of view of their own mental development, as amenable to laws that are passed for the control of an adult population. In the history of the criminal law children and "lunatics" were the first to be exempted from the forms of punishment provided in the statutes. Of course children had to be very young, to begin with, and "lunatics" had to be very "crazy." But this was a beginning, and in the twentieth century this beginning has been acknowledged by incorporation in the juvenile court. One can look forward and visualize a time, in the perhaps not very distant future, when not only will children who are chronologically minors be taken care of entirely in the juvenile courts but those who are psychologically minors will also be cared for in this way. Here again we see an attack upon the old embattled lines of the law and criminal procedure, not a frontal attack but an attack upon the flank. I can imagine many such flank attacks occurring in the next few generations. Our night courts, for example, have only to appreciate that they are dealing with something besides a social problem, that they are dealing with individual human problems that are as much in need of understanding and of individualized treatment as are the children in the juvenile courts; and by and by our criminal courts will see the same light, and ultimately our prisons will be made institutions in which a human being can at least live and preserve his sanity. They are not that now. And at the same time they will become laboratories for the study of human behavior and for its modification along lines of social usefulness.

It will be seen from what has gone before how intimately mental disease becomes related to the law. I have only touched upon some of these relations. It is such relations and many more which are significant from a social point of view that have led to the appreciation of the social aspects of mental disease in their many ramifications. One of these in particular which is a special contribution of this country to the field of psychiatry is the development of the social worker, more specifically the psychiatric social worker. This assistant of the psychiatrist is as important in the field of mental medicine as is the nurse in the field of somatic medicine; and of recent years she has become a very highly trained, highly specialized variety of social worker, not only giving her services to the psychiatrist individually and to the hospital for mental disease, but as psychiatrists are beginning to become permanent adjuncts of criminal courts, as they are beginning to find their way into prisons where they assist the management in dealing with the difficult problems that individual prisoners present, there follows the psychiatric social worker, who hunts up the background of the patient or prisoner as the case may be, who informs the authorities that have to deal with him about this background upon which was erected the disordered conduct which is proving to be such a problem. And finally when the patient is ready for discharge from the hospital she prepares the family for his return home by explaining him and interpreting his behavior to them, and helps him to get a job and to make that exceedingly difficult readjustment that will take him back to society as a useful member.

All these activities involve, however, a concept of the human being which is not an easy one to obtain and which is as difficult to make one's own as in the more definitely biological field is the concept of the organism-as-a-whole. Of this latter concept I will speak more fully later on. But of the concept of the individual as a social unit I will quote some sentences from my paper read at the meeting of the Social Science Research Council in 1927:*

> " If there is any particular definite contribution that American psychiatry has made, it is perhaps along these social lines, and so it is because of these social implications that I believe and psychiatry believes that there is a definite reason for the correlating of the work of the various social sciences and the work of psychiatry.
> " In medicine cellular pathology has been the order of the day for some time. Somatic disease has been explained, by a process of reductive analysis, in terms of the changes that have taken place in the cells of the affected organs as those changes are

* White, W. A.: Psychiatry and the Social Sciences. Amer. Journal of Psychiatry, Vol. 7, No. 5, March, 1928, p. 729.

disclosed by the microscope. The atrophied, disintegrated or otherwise disordered cell has been supposed, at least until recently, to be an adequate explanation of the disordered organ function. With the growing concept of the organism-as-a-whole and the theory of emergent evolution this type of explanation has, to be sure, lost something of its finality, yet we do not fail, because of a change of viewpoint, to continue to interrogate the cell. What is happening is not a complete shift of method and of objective but a revaluation of the place of cellular pathology in the interpretation of pathological processes and its assimilation into the broader concept of the organism-as-a-whole. The gap between organic and functional while probably destined never to be actually closed, is nevertheless constantly narrowing and the two types of explanation run along together with a constantly increasing number of points of contact and correspondingly increasing possibilities of coördination. Despite the new and broader point of view the cell remains not only as important but an indispensable element in the investigations of pathology.

" The social sciences have proceeded in the past largely without a knowledge of the unit components of society, the individuals, because psychology, the science calculated to furnish this knowledge, has in its development been allied with philosophy and morals and has only lately begun to come into recognition as a biological science. If the knowledge of the individual has in the past been acknowledged as desirable this recognition has been for the most part an academic one for as the knowledge did not exist there was nothing of value or substance to mobilize. To have acceded in the past to the general principle that an understanding of the individual was desirable for sociology was largely lip service to a principle which had neither factual data nor a method to support it.

" With the twentieth century, however, psychiatry entered upon an entirely new evaluation of the individual based upon its studies of the mentally diseased, in whom it found uncovered, for the first time, the actual instinctive drives working themselves out under the various impediments and obstacles of the accepted social and cultural standards. It was able to see in mental disease experiments of nature that disclosed the inner structure of the mind as truly as did an accidental wound or the surgeon's knife or the scalpel of the anatomist disclose the structure of the body, and it is this structure, functioning in the living human being, that the psychiatrist is engaged in studying and in trying to understand.

" Many of you probably remember in your school physiologies reading about the Canadian voyageur who had an opening in his stomach and the first observations on digestion were made by this first observation of the interior of the stomach during the ingestion of food. So that in exactly the same way, at least in the same way by analogy, which is a close analogy I think, we see in mental disease the uncovering of certain tendencies in the individual which the average normal man has pretty well snowed under by various protective colorings and devices that render them invisible even to the trained eye.

" Out of his efforts along these lines, he has come to an understanding of much that goes on in the mind under appearances that are no more calculated to disclose the real mechanisms than would the observation of a blacksmith at his forge tell us anything about the neurophysiology of muscular contraction.

" To be sure, in this effort at discovery and formulation speculation, hypothesis and theory are much in evidence as they must needs be in a subject so young in its present form and with such a broad area of borderland in which the visibility is of necessity low. Nevertheless much has already been accomplished and we believe these accomplishments to be of great value to the study of man in his social relations, as reciprocally we believe the accomplishments of the study of socialized man to present much that is illuminating for the understanding of man as an individual.

" The value of a marriage of psychiatry and sociology we may look forward to from the standpoint of a consideration of the social sciences in their relations to the problems of the individual as he emerges. The recently expressed theory of emergent evolution may be briefly stated for our purposes in this way: This theory holds that each new forward integration on the path of evolution emerges into a field of entirely new possibilities which cannot be forecast by the understanding of the previous state. No knowledge of A and B separately will enable us to determine beforehand the history of a partnership relation of A and B, because a third element, an unknown quantity, has been added. The partnership does not consist of two components, A and B, but of three, A and B and the relation between them. This partnership, in the language of emergent evolution, would be an emergent, to all intents and purposes a new being with laws of action unpredictable on the basis of the preceding lower stage of development. The higher can never be fully explained by the lower, and it might seem that I was herein contradicting what I have thus far said that seemed to point in that direction. For example, life will not receive its explanation in chemistry because in the chemical compounds there is no life and one cannot expect to find an explanation for life where it does not exist, and so in all of the higher emergences, the explanation never will be full and complete by reductive analysis because by the mere reduction the very integration which it is sought to explain ceases to exist.

" But to revert to the analogy to cellular pathology. If we examine the blood we will find the cells of which it is composed so characteristic that they are unmistakable, even though we find them under the microscope without knowing their source. The same might be said of other cells from other parts of the body, and no histologist would ever confuse a section of kidney and a section from a voluntary muscle. So that while from this philosophical point of view the higher contains the lower and can never be interpreted in terms of the lower altogether because it contains more than the lower, still the understanding of both levels must go hand in hand. While it is true that we never could explain the purpose that lay in the mind of the blacksmith as he pounded his anvil by any examination of the cellular components of his voluntary muscle, it is also true that we could not have a full understanding of how that purpose could be brought to pass without such information. The value, then, of a marriage of psychiatry and sociology we look forward to from the standpoint of society as an emergent and the general philosophical attitude of the interpretation of the lower by the higher in the scheme of evolution as offering much to us as psychiatrists in the understanding of man's individual heritage as it comes to him in the precipitated traditions and mores of the herd. Here, if I see aright, we have a reciprocal relationship—man, society—neither element of which can be safely ignored if we are to understand the other. The study of man is, after all, only a study of natural forces operating in smaller dimensions than they operate in in society; and the analytic method of science which would carry the study of the interpretation of man to his cellular components would be another step in the direction of still smaller dimensions, as would the still further step which carried the study into the realm of chemistry. From this point of view, therefore, the study of the individual by the psychiatrist and of society by the sociologist present problems that lie in different dimensions though not necessarily dealing with different forces.

"Man, as the psychiatrist sees him, although he presents infinite differences, is from the very beginning fundamentally much more like his fellows than different from them. His original equipment is very similar if not identical in each instance, but as soon as it begins to function the infinite play of stimulus and reaction begins at once to produce those kaleidoscopic changes which differentiate each one from his fellow, and the longer he lives and the more complicated become his relations the more different he seems to be although fundamentally he remains the same. These differences, however, work themselves out in society, and it does not seem possible to understand their social manifestations unless we have some knowledge of their individual nature and origin."

It will be seen from the above quotations that I conceive that here we have the basis for the coming into existence of what is beginning to be known as a social psychiatry, which deals with man as a social being in his relations to his fellows and is primarily interested not only in the problems presented by the dependent, defective and delinquent classes but in a host of other aspects of man in his social relations. Religion, education, economics, in fact every activity of man as a social animal, will have to come to a certain " transvaluation of values " as a result of the information which the psychiatrist is rapidly accumulating about man as he studies him with his more intimate and refined methods, particularly as he sees him mentally ill and with his motives disclosed to full view. These are some of the directions in which psychiatry is heading up as a result of its renaissance in the twentieth century.

# CHAPTER XII

## ADVANCES ALONG MANY FRONTS

The thirteenth has been called the greatest of centuries. I have often wondered whether those that follow us when they get as far away from the present day as we are away from the thirteenth century may not possibly, in looking back over the record of man's accomplishments, come to the conclusion that the twentieth was the greatest of centuries; for, if the reader has not already divined it, let me specify more definitely at this point that practically all of the great advances that I have been recording and am still to record in the following pages had their inception at the beginning of the present century. It is true that the beginnings were often inconspicuous, as beginnings have a habit of being, but as we look back over the record we find that that is what happened.

I have already recorded a number of these beginnings which have blossomed out into full-blown and well recognized movements, and I have indicated that to my mind the present era might well be designated the scientific period in the historical sequence of events in the care of the so-called " insane," as designating the general spirit of these many advances and as differentiating it from the previous period, the humanitarian period, during which great effort was expended upon getting the " insane " out of prisons and poor-houses, accumulating them in state hospitals, building for their accommodation, arranging for their care—not only their physical care but their care as sick people, and also making the necessary arrangements, economic, legislative and administrative, to carry out the requirements for their care.

I have already said something of the development of the psychopathic hospital. I have told of the beginning of this idea as it expressed itself in Pavilion F at the Albany Hospital. It was already existent but unrecognized as such in the Psychopathic Pavilion at Bellevue Hospital, New York City. Then there followed the building of the Psychopathic Hospital at Boston in connection with the buildings of the Harvard Medical School, where it was planned that this institution should function not only as a psychopathic hospital but as a teaching adjunct of the University. This institution was devised and directed in its early days by that outstanding character in American psychiatry, Dr. E. E. Southard, perhaps one of the most unique characters in psychiatry and one of the most productive that have been developed in this country. His untimely death in 1920 left unfinished many works on which he was engaged. He was followed in his Directorship of the Psychopathic Hospital by the present incumbent, Dr. C. Macfie Campbell. Then there was the Psychopathic Hospital at Ann Arbor, Michigan, also connected with the State University and which was brought into existence largely by the efforts of that energetic and farseeing gentleman, Dr. W. J. Herdman, whose position as Director since his death has been occupied by the eminent American psychiatrist, Dr. Albert M. Barrett. As is usual in such situations, the Director is also the Professor of Psychiatry in the University. Then there came the Phipps Clinic in connection with the Johns Hopkins Hospital, in Baltimore, to which Dr. Adolf Meyer was called from his position at the Pathological Institute of the New York State Hospitals, which had moved from its palatial quarters on Madison Avenue to Wards Island. If it were my purpose to dwell upon the personalities of American psychiatrists for the past forty years I should have to stop here and elaborate at considerable length. In many respects Dr. Meyer has been the outstanding influence in the development of psychiatry in this country for about forty years, and practically no major enterprise has been projected in the field of psychiatry which he has not influenced in some way. Then there is the Psychopathic Pavilion at Denver, Colorado, with Dr. Franklin G. Ebaugh as its Director, also associated with the University, in this case the University of Colorado. Dr. Ebaugh is rapidly making his impression upon American psychiatry as a result of his development in the field of teaching, and also, particularly, by his introduction of the psychiatrist to the wards devoted to general medical cases.

To leave the matter of psychopathic pavilions at this point, I may add that the development of psychopathic wards in general hospitals, particularly in municipal hospitals, is coming to be a recognized part of the scheme of such institutions. For example, there is the Psychopathic Ward connected with the Municipal Hospital of Buffalo, New York, which was provided in the original plans and specifications and incorporated in the main body of the hospital as a result of the efforts of my good friend, Dr. Herman G. Matzinger, Professor of Psychiatry in the School of Medicine of the University of Buffalo, since deceased. An interesting story about this clinic is, after all, very much more than a story. It really is typical of the experience in this field of endeavor. It seems that with the completion of the arrangements for incorporating a psychopathic ward in this hospital the timid and the conservative individuals were naturally apprehensive of what might result, but they very modestly expressed themselves in the warning that in all probability the noise that would emanate from the psychopathic ward would be very disturbing to the wards immediately adjacent, especially those wards in the wings which ran parallel to the wing in which the psychopathic ward was located and which were separated therefrom by only a few feet. After the wards were occupied the real thing that happened was not that the adjacent wards found fault with the noise of the psychopathic patients but that the psychopathic patients found fault with the noise that issued from the adjoining obstetrical wards. An equally illuminating story comes to me from another source. The psychopathic ward in a general hospital was put in charge of an able psychiatrist, and, although I am drawing somewhat upon my imagination, I nevertheless can see in my mind's eye the medical staff of that hospital standing around, as it were, and looking this psychiatrist over and wondering after all what sort of an animal he was and what he was going to do, because the general practitioner and the medical specialist know very little about the psychiatrist and his functions. At any rate, they kept hands off and waited and watched, and they saw patients coming into his wards and going out again and after all nothing very serious happening, nothing in fact that was very unusual. That was the remarkable part of it. And because he was there and they saw him every day, psychiatry, though they did not know very much about it and what it was, was necessarily presented to their minds frequently, and from time to time one of their patients would present symptoms that even the most obtuse practitioner would recognize as mental—at least he would know that there was somebody right at his elbow who constantly reminded him that there were such things as mental symptoms. Also, under these circumstances, the psychiatrist was occasionally called in consultation and occasionally as a result patients were transferred from other departments of the hospital to the psychopathic ward. Gradually the staff became acquainted. They discovered that the psychiatrist was a man of at least reasonable intelligence and that apparently he had had some medical education and experience, and so the day came when one of the physicians of his own motion transferred a patient to the psychopathic ward with a diagnosis of " mental " and with a record that showed that nothing had been disclosed upon the physical side. Now the psychiatrist received this patient in due course and undertook to examine him to find out what the trouble was, and lo and behold, he uncovered evidences of physical disorder that had escaped the observation of the internist, whereupon he returned the patient to the internist with his diagnosis. Had the internist or the rest of the staff of this hospital been narrow-minded and vindictive and jealous they might only have had these qualities in their personality make-up aroused, but fortunately they were not and the net result of this experience was a great rise in the stock of the psychiatrist. He was recognized at once as being a doctor, a real doctor who had been through the medical mill just like the rest of them, who actually recognized physical disease when it existed and did not call it by some psychopathological name. And so he began to be called more and more into consultation and he became an accepted member of the staff, in fact as well as in name, and psychiatry through his influence has become recognized in this hospital as one of the essential activities of the institution.

After all, it is really amazing how blind people are to the things they are not looking for, and how this experience that I have illustrated by these two stories repeats itself in one form or another over and over again. Another story I have in mind is the story of an eminent cardiologist who was taking a psychiatrist through his wards, and when he comes to the bedside of a patient with cardiac decompensation he tells the psychiatrist that this is the third or the fourth time that this patient has been in the hospital for this same reason, and that after two or three or four weeks rest in bed he will probably be all right and go out again. And when the psychiatrist asks the cardiologist what this man's business is the cardiologist does not know. As a matter of fact, he was a piano mover and he was permitted to come into the hospital with a cardiac decompensation and then go out of the hospital and go back to his job of carrying pianos on his back up and down stairs until he decompensated again, without a word of warning of any sort. Of course many stories like this could be told, but I will hasten forward.

The psychopathic ward in general hospitals, as I have said, has become a well recognized unit of such institutions. And aside from Buffalo I might mention the very excellently conducted Psychopathic Ward of the Henry Ford Hospital, of Detroit, which has as its Chief of Staff my friend, Dr. Thomas J. Heldt. Similar developments are occurring also in slightly divergent directions, such as, for example, the work that Dr. George S. Stevenson is doing in connection with the gastrointestinal division of the Cornell Clinic, where he has gradually been enabled to uncover the psychopathic components in many gastrointestinal types of disorder.

To leave this aspect of the subject, for the present at least, and turn again to the question of juvenile courts and delinquency, no discussion of this subject should fail to note the beginnings of this enterprise in Chicago, with Judge Julian W. Mack on the Bench and Dr. William Healy as the Psychiatrist. This set-up, in particular Dr. Healy's position, was made possible by that wise, public-spirited, and far-seeing Mrs. Ethel S. Dummer of that city. The net result of the work accomplished was a definite impression upon the concept of delinquency, from both the legal and the medical side, which has had much to do with the whole development in this country ever since. Dr. Healy fortunately was very productive and reduced his experiences to writing rapidly where others could consult them. Judge Mack was humanitarian at heart and was never bound by the futile traditions of the law. In talking with me upon one occasion and in discussing the frequency with which he was approached by interested parties, particularly parents whose children were then before his Court—even to the extent that in riding downtown on the cars they often came in and sat next to him to tell him about their boys, he said to me that he never repulsed any of these approaches, that so far as he was concerned he never could learn too much about these youngsters. How wholesome an attitude, and how different from that of the judge who ordinarily will not listen to a single thing anybody says to him except someone who is officially privileged to speak in the court during its session, on the theory that he is afraid his mind will become prejudiced. In the same proceeding, however, lawyers say all sorts of impossible things before the jury, which are stricken out of the record by the Court on the theory that striking them out makes them as if they never had existed; and yet everybody knows that this is not so and the lawyers use this subterfuge for getting incompetent matters before the jury. The old regidities of the law which have resulted in a trial becoming a mere form in which technical details are more important than facts, have been seriously challenged by the juvenile court with such an attitude as that indicated by the above story.

One can not dismiss the subject of the relation of psychiatry to the criminal law without mentioning the Massachusetts law requiring the examination of certain felons previous to their trial. This law went into effect in September, 1921, and is sometimes known as the Briggs law because of the great personal activity and influence of Dr. L. Vernon Briggs in bringing it to pass. The original form of this law* is as follows:

> " Whenever a person is indicted by a grand jury for a capital offense or whenever a person, who is known to have been indicted for any other offense more than once or to have been previously convicted of a felony, is indicted by a grand jury or bound over for trial in the superior court, the clerk of the court in which the indictment is returned, or the clerk of the district court or the trial justice, as the case may be, shall give notice to the department of mental diseases, and the department shall cause such person to be examined with a view to determine his mental condition and the existence of any mental disease or defect which would affect his criminal responsibility. The department shall file a report of its investigation with the clerk of the court in which the trial is to be held, and the report shall be accessible to the court, the district attorney, and to the attorney for the accused, and shall be admissible as evidence of the mental condition of the accused."

Reports have been made of progress under the operation of this statute and up to the present writing those reports are exceedingly favorable. They indicate that very much has been accomplished in the recognition of psychotic and defective individuals and much assistance given to the courts in the handling of this type of cases and their differentiation from the general group of offenders. Incidentally the courts learn a great deal about the concepts of the psychiatrist and come to have a much better understanding of human behavior as they meet it in their courts, and, like the juvenile courts, so this law functions to undermine and dissipate the old hide-bound traditions of criminal procedure.

In conformity with the results of the mental hygiene movement, which in its efforts to improve the care of the " insane " finally came to undertaking to outline a mental hygiene that would at least help to prevent mental disease, and in doing so found that it had to go back earlier and earlier in the life of the individual in order to apply this hygiene effectively, there have arisen in recent years the so-called child guidance clinics, which undertake to tackle the problem of maladjustment and its inception in childhood, scotch it there as it were, and so prevent forever its development into those major disturbances

---

*Cited by Glueck, S. Sheldon, in Mental Disorder and the Criminal Law. Boston: Little, Brown & Co., 1925, p. 58.

that afflict the individual in later life. These mental hygiene clinics were developed not primarily to undertake either the problem of the defective child or of the delinquent child but they were devised for the purpose of helping to solve the difficulties presented by the problem child, and, of course, as every child is more or less a problem, to assist in the unfoldment and understanding of an adequate approach to the whole field of raising children in a way to insure as far as possible a well balanced mind. These child guidance clinics were sponsored and financed by the Commonwealth Fund and were set up in a number of the larger cities throughout the United States, not arbitrarily but at the request of these several cities, with the understanding that they would be maintained for a certain period of time until the experiment was well under way and it could be evaluated, and after that the cities would take them over, maintain them and budget them. This experimental period passed some years ago and in order that the results that were attained should not be lost, that the work might be properly integrated and to a certain extent a parent institution should oversee it and exercise a certain amount of direction to prevent individual institutions widely separated from others of their kind from going off at tangents, a Child Guidance Institute was set up in New York City, which had as its principal function teaching and research. This has been in existence now for several years but owing to the financial stringency, which has affected the great foundations as well as the individual, it is going to be necessary to close it during the coming year.

These child guidance clinics formed important affiliations in their several municipalities, not only with medical men on the one hand and psychologists on the other, but more particularly with the educational system and with such organizations as the parent-teachers associations and the like, and in each instance where they have functioned they have become quite important centers of activity along the lines of their special interests and also centers of influence and helpfulness. The child guidance clinics give some idea of the extent to which psychiatric ideals have departed, or one might better say have expanded, from the original nucleus of the state hospital, in this instance into exceedingly significant extra-mural activities. Perhaps no better idea could be gathered as to how far this movement of extra-mural psychiatry has gone than to indicate for a moment the extent to which it is represented in psychiatric clinics throughout the country. These clinics have been growing in number and significance for a number of years, and in 1925 the Commonwealth Fund issued a Directory of such clinics. At that time the total number recorded was 318. Three years later, 1928, they found it necessary to get out another Directory, in which the number of clinics recorded was 492; whereas the last Directory, published in 1931, showed that this number had increased to 674. These clinics, naturally, are of all degrees of excellence. Some of them serve children only, some adults only, some of them are on a part-time basis, a not inconsiderable number are on a full-time basis, and, of the 674, 232 provide the three-fold service of psychiatrist, psychologist and psychiatric social worker. It is of significance, too, that many of these clinics are maintained by the state hospitals. In Massachusetts, particularly, the general principle has been accepted that the state hospital has a certain responsibility for the territory from which it draws; and as the psychiatric social worker has been added to the state hospital staff and has become interested in helping to place the discharged patients satisfactorily and assist them in making a readjustment on their return to their home environment, so it soon became evident that many former patients who felt themselves slipping, and many others who never had been patients but who were experiencing certain danger signals, sought the advice of these state hospital representatives, and therefore it came about as a natural sequel almost that the state hospital should establish clinics in some of the more important centers of population within their districts and that a physician from the state hospital should journey to these clinics, say once a week, and see the various people who needed advice and help. This principle and this method has extended in a number of directions, and many of the state hospitals now maintain such extra-mural centers of helpfulness in their corresponding districts. What effect the depression has had upon the number, extent and personnel of all these clinics I do not know. I fear, naturally, that their activities may be somewhat contracted as a result of it.

Along with these rather extensive developments that have reached far outside the confines of the state hospital, there have gone along equally significant changes within. I have already mentioned the development of nursing care. This, as a matter of fact, started before the beginning of the century, but it did not get well under way until the opening years of nineteen hundred. It was easy enough to recognize that our employees needed training, and we proceeded to give it to them along the lines of instruction that were given to nurses in training in general hospitals. This corresponded to the general tendency of these early days to turn the state hospital into a

general hospital in its methods of procedure. As the years have gone
on, however, the element of error in this concept has become more
and more evident, and it has come to be realized that the mental
nurse needs a training very considerably different from the training
given the general nurse; and in fact our attitude with reference to
the training of nurses is coming to be very much like that with reference to the training of physicians, namely, that the mental aspect of
disease should receive much more consideration in the training of
both groups. At any rate, the training schools developed. In the State
of New York, for example, they came under the immediate supervision of the State Department of Education. In other institutions,
especially the well endowed private institutions, an already trained
nurse graduated from a general hospital was brought into the institution and there expected to get her special experience with mental
disease. This scheme, in my experience, has never worked very well.
The nurse trained in a general hospital who has no systematic training in the care of mental diseases is often a good deal of a liability
in a mental hospital. She is all very well in getting ready for an
operation but she may be everlastingly blind to all of the more important aspects of her duty as relates directly to the care of mental
patients. And so through the years it has naturally come to pass that
there have grown up in these institutions training schools which are
meeting the standards of the training schools in general hospitals,
sending their nurses to other institutions to affiliate in such subjects
as children's diseases and obstetrics, clinical instruction in which
naturally is not available in a state hospital, and then giving them that
special training in mental disease nursing which makes them valuable
to the mental institution, and so graduating them as trained nurses in
fact and in accordance with the standards required by the National
League of Nursing Education and yet at the same time equipping
them for the special work of the mental hospital. Even in these days
of depression when the general hospitals are doing away with their
training schools, the mental hospitals have had to keep their training
schools in operation wherever possible because there is no source of
supply for mental nurses as there is for general nurses. Then again,
of course the very great value of having teaching in the institution
is something which is perhaps more significant in a state hospital than
in a general hospital, because in the latter all of the resident physicians are internes and are on their way to private practice or to some
special activity that will take them away from the hospital in a few
months, whereas in the state hospital with its permanent resident

staff it is essential that a stimulus like teaching should be maintained wherever and as long as possible.

Another one of the additions to the personnel of the hospital which have come to be accepted as standard equipment is the occupational aide. Occupation, as I have already indicated, always was an important factor in planning for the care and treatment of institutionalized patients, and I repeat that I wonder frequently whether the old methods of teaching the patients to work on the farm can be very much improved upon; yet a great many patients are not reached by methods that are so crude as those employed in the old days, and so from the early days of the century there has been a growing sentiment in favor of the occupational aide and she has come to the hospital, introduced her workshop, in some instances on the wards where she wishes to reach the patients who have not enough initiative to go to work outside and in other instances she has been provided with a special occupational building or a series of rooms. In any case, the patients have been more largely occupied. This is very productive. They have made a great many beautiful things that have sales value and their interest has been ensnared by the work to their advantage and increased happiness. Like many other things that have happened in the state hospitals in the last quarter century, it is difficult to evaluate occupational therapy. Nobody would like to go without it and yet to specifically relate it to the net results that are obtained does not seem to be by any means an easy task. One thing that it does, however, is that it helps to effect a change in the personnel of the institution. It brings in a group of technically highly equipped, intelligent young women, as a rule, and this group added to the hospital personnel tends to raise the average throughout. It has always been a good thing when some new device has brought into the hospital a superior group of personnel. Occupational therapy has been one of those devices, and although this is not one of the results with which it is usually accredited but is a result indirectly traceable to the use of the occupational aide, still to my mind it is by no means of minor importance.

The same thing exactly happened with the introduction of the trained nurse. A higher group of caretakers was brought into the hospital which brought along with it higher standards, which translated themselves into a general rise of the average level of the personnel throughout the institution, which meant more intelligent appreciation of the problems of the hospital and more specifically of the problems of the individual patient and a greater ability to coöperate with the management understandingly in their solution.

A somewhat similar state of affairs maintains with respect to the introduction of hydrotherapy, although here the net improvement in conditions is probably not so much dependent on the personnel in this department as upon the therapeutic value of the method and the fact that as a substitute for sedative drugs it became a means by which it was possible to discard them so that now sedatives and hypnotics are reduced to a minimum, disturbed conditions are recognized for the most part as being acute and transient and are adequately cared for by some type of hydrotherapy, of which the continuous bath is a very important adjunct.

Not dissimilar in its indirect effects, such as I have indicated with reference to the occupational aide and the trained nurse, has been the introduction of the dietitian into the hospital personnel. This has insured scientifically controlled dietaries for patients. It has enabled the hospital to put into effect special dietaries for special diseases, such as diabetes, nephritis, various disorders of metabolism, etc., which could hardly have been done under the old regime, and, further, as with the occupational aide, it has introduced a high grade type of individual into the personnel. The dietitian has had a long education and experience. She is not infrequently a college graduate who has taken special instruction in dietetics. And so we have another instance of the bringing into the institution of a highly intelligent group, a small group, to be sure, but one which necessarily has its general effect upon the functioning of the hospital as a whole.

What I have said about the occupational aides and the dietitians and their effect upon the personnel of the state hospital needs to be elaborated just a little bit in order to give the full picture. The general results of the raising of the standard of the personnel by the introduction of the three groups discussed, namely, the trained nurse, the occupational aide and the dietitian, have been merely outstanding instances of what has happened from the top to the bottom of the state hospital. The standard of educational requirements, of technical equipment, of character all along the line has been gradually on the upward trend. In addition to the groups that I have mentioned there have come into the institution the technicians who work in the laboratory in connection with the cutting and staining of sections and in the X-ray department in connection with the taking of X-ray pictures and their development, the laboratorians who perform the usual technique for obtaining clinical specimens, blood, sputum, etc., and make the routine examinations of these specimens. All along the line the work has become more technical, it has required greater preparation in order to do it, with a resulting rise in the standard of

the people who are employed in the various capacities. It is interesting in this connection to note that each one of these groups is very
apt to get the idea that all of the improvement that has taken place in
the state hospital is due to its particular efforts. The occupational
aide is sure that she has introduced a revolutionary measure into the
state hospital around which have developed all of the great improvements which have taken place; the trained nurse is equally sure
from her point of view that she has done the same thing. And so it
goes, but when one sits down and calmly contemplates all these
developments he feels sure, not only that they are all wrong but that
they are all right. What really has happened is that improvement in
institutional care has been the net result of all of these agencies.
Each one of them has contributed its bit and I know of no way of
untangling this complicated skein and sorting out just how much
and what has come from each source.

There is one other agency that ought not to go unmentioned in
the development of a great mental hospital, and that is the library.
There are naturally two divisions of any adequate library equipment—the division which deals especially with the medical and scientific works and periodicals, and the division which deals with the
circulating library devoted to furnishing books, magazines, news-
papers and reading matter generally to the patient population. The
former I will not speak of in this place. The latter I will only mention to state that it has become in my opinion one of the essential
components of hospital organization and that if I were to pick out
the outstanding fact that it teaches us as we watch its operation I
would say that it has taught us what we have learned over and over
again, perhaps, from other points of view, namely, that the so-called
" insane " and the so-called normal person are not fundamentally
different. The patients in these institutions read almost precisely,
if not quite precisely, the same literature that the average citizen reads
outside. We have had our circulation carefully reduced to per-
centages and compared it with the similar classification of the circulation of the Carnegie Library in Washington and they are practically
identical. We not only learn that the mentally ill and the mentally
well are much closer together than most people like to think, but we
learn the futility of all the censorship schemes which many librarians
have launched to prevent mentally ill patients from getting hold of
literature that will do them harm, a point of view which I am sure is
based 99 per cent upon a myth.

# CHAPTER XIII

## EXTRA-MURAL DEVELOPMENTS

Perhaps no single feature in the advance of psychiatry has been more characteristic than its escape from the confines of the state hospital and its development along many lines of extra-mural activity. I have already briefly discussed the mental hygiene movement. Although this movement originated with a desire to improve conditions within the state hospital it did not long confine itself to such objectives and today " mental hygiene " is a term that is well known by the laity. It is so well known, in fact, that any public meeting that puts on a mental hygiene program will almost without exception be crowded to the doors, so eager are the people to learn about this mind of theirs, something about how it works and something about how it gets them into trouble and how to prevent such trouble. A knowledge of the mind has seemed to exert a peculiar fascination upon the people, so that the various aspects of psychology are receiving wide notice. The psychological novel is a well known development in the literary field, and all sorts of books have issued in the past few years that have been prompted by the mental hygiene movement and by the disclosures which have been made by psychoanalysis.

One of the important directions in which these interests have manifested themselves is in connection with the great educational institutions and departments. In attempting to develop a mental hygiene program that would be for mental disease what preventive medicine has heretofore been for somatic disease, that would include the problems of mental disease as a part of a great public health program, I have already indicated that it became necessary to seek further and further back in the life of the individual for the factors that finally got him into trouble. In the course of this search naturally the school period came under scrutiny so that as a logical consequence psychiatrists sought to see what could be accomplished with the student body itself in the great educational institutions. Psychiatrists were taken on the medical staffs of some of the larger universities, and it soon became evident that there was plenty of work for them to do. In the first place, the students themselves had their own personal difficulties, which in many instances were great, and just so soon as there was a psychiatrist who was prepared to discuss these difficulties with them intelligently and who was free from the necessity of reporting his findings to the faculty—because the keeping of information confidential is an important aspect of all psychiatric contacts, they literally flocked to him for help. The result was what might be expected. A college boy is in the adolescent period of his existence, when the primitive instincts are battling for expression and when he himself has as yet frequently not developed character traits of sufficient strength so that he can count upon keeping them in suppression. The result naturally is disastrous in many instances, and many students develop frank mental disease, others commit suicide and still others enter upon delinquent careers. This condition of affairs had never really been known before. Infractions of discipline were met by various punishments, and failure to pass examinations by dismissal. Students who did not make adjustments were gotten rid of in one way and another, and the great problem of the mental difficulties such as I have indicated never really seeped through to the attention of the authorities in any adequate form. Now all this was changed. The student began to be understood. He was assisted with his difficulties, and in many instances the teaching staff of the university was assisted to understand him. His failures in class were often found to be due to removable conditions, so that it was not necessary to drop him from the rolls but only to correct these conditions, which very frequently naturally centered about the home. And so there was gained a whole new point of view of the college student and of his problems, which in the last analysis was mutually helpful to him and to the authorities of the university.

This development in the mental hygiene of students came along at a happy time because contemporaneously there was the development of an attempt to evaluate the student psychologically by mental tests, not to say also the attempt to guide him in the direction he should go as a result of information disclosed by these tests. So in this way the whole problem of education has received enlightenment, particularly because the light has come from an increased knowledge of the properties of the individuals who are to be educated.

This movement did not stop at the college because it was found that many students entering college were already badly handicapped, and so we find the psychiatrist seeking out the solution of his problem in the preparatory schools and finally in the primary schools. Private schools have seen the light and have also moved in the same direction.

And finally the psychiatrist is sought for by the educational institution itself, not primarily to look after the mental health of the students but primarily to study the problems, the mechanisms, of the whole educational proceeding, its subject matter, the method of its presentation, etc. Recently, for example, a psychiatrist, Dr. Frederick L. Patry, has been taken on by the New York State Department of Education. This is an indication of the extent to which psychiatry is finding its expression in one of the most important activities of the state.

This is an example of how psychiatry has been coming out of its nineteenth century shell, emerging into extra-mural activities. I have already mentioned a number of others: the advent of the psychiatrist as a permanent fixture in the functioning of the criminal courts and in the work of the juvenile courts: the development of the psychiatric social worker and the growth of schools which give her adequate training: the growth and development of psychiatric clinics, those connected with the state hospitals and those connected with other institutions and those that are independent, the child guidance clinics and the habit clinics, which I have not as yet mentioned, which are for the purpose of dealing with the problems of very young children: the development of psychiatry as a specialty represented by psychiatrists in practice along with the other medical specialties, and in this field we have the psychiatrist in the usual sense of that term; we find the psychiatrist who specializes in court work, and in recent years we find a gradually increasing number of psychoanalysts: the development of more elaborate teaching in the field of medical psychology, psychopathology and clinical psychiatry and psychotherapy in the medical schools, so as to equip the average medical student with the fundamental principles of mental medicine as he has been equipped for generations in the fundamental principles of anatomy and physiology so that he might understand the functioning of the body; and the ever-increasing demand upon the psychiatrist for public lectures and courses of instruction in various departments of his specialty, particularly in mental hygiene programs, parent-teachers programs and also before general medical groups—all of which testifies to the increasing interest in this department of medicine and to the extraordinary change that has taken place since the practice of psychiatry was confined within the walls of the state hospital. These are the main movements, of which naturally many variants and minor expressions will be found here and there. There

are the health surveys that are made from time to time and which
now are very apt to include a psychiatrist and a program which will
consider mental as well as physical health, such surveys, for example,
as were made of the prisons of the country only about four years ago.
We have similar surveys for geographical districts, of groups of
unemployed, of different types of institutions, etc.  We have child
psychology being developed as a special branch of psychology along
experimental lines, as is taking place at Yale under the influence and
leadership of Dr. Arnold Gesell and which is adding its quota of
information to the general knowledge of psychology as it comes from
this genetic field.  There are clinical psychologists who started some
years ago largely to make intelligence tests but who have developed
a great number of psychological measuring devices for various
aspects of the personality and now undertake to study in this way
some of the complex problems the personality presents.  Some of
these clinical psychologists advise as to vocation and some of them
go so far as to undertake actual therapeutic work.  The well equipped
clinical psychologist is beginning to find her way into the large hospitals and into the various clinics and also into the prisons and courts,
working along with the psychiatrist and supplying particularly that
type of information which indicates, usually in terms of psychological
age or intellectual quotient, the limitations of the given individual in
certain directions and his special capacities in other directions, so that
a general survey of his personality has this additional light thrown
upon his assets and liabilities.

Last, but not least, there is the development in industrial psychiatry.  The so-called hard-headed business man is not presumed to
invest his capital in wild and unproductive schemes.  He is anxious
that there should be an adequate return upon every investment he
makes.  And so it might be some indication as to the importance that
psychiatry has come to assume that large business enterprises that
employ considerable numbers of people are now calling upon the
psychiatrist to help them in their problems.  Business in this country
has had a history that is something like the history of the pioneer.
In the early days the pioneer cut down all the trees he wanted to build
his house, and what he did not use could lie and rot and no harm was
done.  The supply of trees was practically infinite.  But as the
country has grown and the border of advancing industry has swept
further and further across the country, the forests have been invaded
more and more until now the conservation of forests has become one

of the major problems of government. So the early industries, without competition, conducted their affairs in a wasteful way, but now that every industry meets keen competition it is necessary to take account of every bit of lost motion and try to eliminate it. So it has come to be understood that the taking in of an employee and keeping him for an indefinite period of time, sometimes for several years, and then suddenly discharging him because of some technical infraction of a rule, was a very expensive proposition. The firm has too much invested in him to be able to indulge in such wasteful procedures. It was equally wasteful to spend six or eight or ten months in training a person to do a certain job which a little previous examination would indicate that he never could do—all that training, all that expenditure of money, time and labor would be lost. So the psychiatrist has gone in to try to straighten out these problems, to try to weed out the applicants that can not be utilized from those that can be. Then, having developed a plan for doing this sort of thing, he has been asked further to take up the problem of promotions and innumerable other personal problems of the great mass of employees, until nowadays the psychiatrist and the psychologist have been brought into the plant to study methods of production, to see whether production can not be increased by a better understanding of the psychological situation and a better adjustment of the individual to his job. All of these things show the growing importance of psychiatry, and, also, this development of industrial psychiatry shows how far flung are psychiatric interests from those of the state hospital of the nineteenth century.

For some time many of us have been feeling that psychiatry, generally speaking, usually as expressed by mental hygiene, was oversold, by which we meant that the demands that were made upon it exceeded the possibilities of adequate response owing to the fact that there was not sufficient well-trained personnel to undertake the various problems that we are being asked to help solve. This is one of the reasons, perhaps the principal reason, why the increased pressure has been brought upon medical schools for additional hours in the curriculum devoted to the study of mind. The extreme picture, therefore, of the nineteenth century and the present day amounts to about this: that whereas the old insane asylum was held under suspicion and in awe, and patients were not sent there except as a last resort and then every conceivable iniquity was believed to occur behind its walls, today psychiatry and the psychiatrist are received with open arms in almost every direction and asked to help solve the problems of almost everybody. Of course the change has not been complete in every direction. Many of the old superstitions still exist although they are not so prominent, but let something a little unusual arise that calls in question the excellence of the local institution and it would seem that all of them suddenly bob up their heads with renewed vigor and act as if nothing had ever happened to them. Aside from these instances, however, this very radical change has been taking place very rapidly through the years in the direction which I have indicated.

# CHAPTER XIV

## THE MIND COMES INTO ITS OWN—MEANING REPLACES
### DESCRIPTION

I have already indicated that in the nineteenth century psychology was still closely allied with philosophy and ethics, or what was then called " moral philosophy," and has had a hard time to substantiate its right to a place with the biological sciences. It is probably as difficult to make a modern student understand the status of thought regarding the mind which existed some forty years ago as it is to make the modern interne understand the conditions that prevailed in the old asylum of the same period. Just as the removal of restraint, physical and chemical, from the armamentarium of the asylum has resulted in there being no patients who need restraint, so the change of point of view regarding psychological phenomena has made equally unnecessary certain necessities of description and definition which were felt to be basic in the old days. And in the new world of thought that has developed under these changes people who live today find themselves unable to translate the events of yesterday into understandable experiences. We can not very well feel ourselves into situations from which and out of which we have developed. Nevertheless the thing that has happened in this realm is of the utmost significance to psychiatry, and it is so recent in its occurrence that there is some chance that everyone may have passed through similar stages of development.

In the first place, man has had a mind ever since man has existed, but it is only in very recent times that mental phenomena as such have attracted his attention. Mental phenomena perhaps have been so obvious that they have escaped perception, but what we are fighting for now, namely, the recognition that mental facts have a reality quite as much as do any others, was in those days accepted without, however, the appreciation that these realities were mental. If a man saw a ghost there never was any question about such a phenomenon being psychological in origin or, as we should say today, psychogenic. He accepted the fact of the ghost and believed in it. The philosophers, however, have for a long time been worrying about the nature of the mind. They have been trying to define its relations to the body. This interesting proceeding has been going on for centuries, with how much result I do not know,—but very little, apparently, that is of any use to us today. Mind during all these centuries of recorded history has been the great mystery of the universe, and man has failed always before in his efforts at its solution; but in that respect man has not failed any more completely than he has with reference to many other ultimate problems. He never has been able to tell exactly what gravity was, or, for that matter, electricity, or even matter itself. He has always failed to answer these ultimate questions in the clear-cut terms of a definition, which he seems to be always seeking but never able to find. But the last century was bent upon continuing the search, while the present century has for the most part abandoned it as useless. We may take our lesson from Newton, who perhaps was quite as unable to define gravity as any of us but who nevertheless was able to formulate the law in accordance with which gravity, whatever it is in essence, works. The psychologist and the psychiatrist are equally incapable of telling what mind is but they can tell some of the ways in which it works, some of the things that it does. And so instead of wasting our time in attempting to define the indefinable and describe the indescribable, we are now bent on trying to answer the questions of how and when and why events come about. We are trying to read meaning into the phenomenon as we see it and realizing meantime that the test of science is the capacity to predict.

These changes in the way of thinking about mental phenomena came to pass, probably, for many reasons and not as a result of any one particular cause. However, it would appear that the old method of description which resulted in a static psychology had about used itself up and further progress with the old ideas as guides had become pretty near impossible. On the other hand, similar changes of viewpoint were happening all along the line, in every direction, and so presumably this change in the way in which psychological phenomena were thought about is probably only a part of the great change in the way in which man was coming to think of the cosmos and all of his relations to it and its relations to him. The Bergsonian philosophy, which was essentially dynamic, helped this movement considerably in this country, as did also the psychoanalytic movement more specifically, while the growth of different tendencies in psychology, more particularly the growth of the Gestalt psychology, added their quota of influence. From the beginning of the nineteenth century, when the mind was considered an inexplicable phenomenon and was described in the most simple and naïve way in the average text-book and had little or no place in the general scheme of the cosmos except perhaps in the thoughts of the theologian, when it was left out of account entirely by the biologist and the physician excluded it from his thinking although in reality he necessarily dealt with its phenomena, the more successfully the more intuitively, and even the psychiatrist had the most indefinite, simplistic, childlike concept of this most significant and most complex phenomenon, I suspect of the entire universe so far as I know—psychological events were not given meaning, and for the most part the possibility of their having any meaning was not even vaguely suspected. So that our patients did this, that or the other thing without fitting into any scheme except the crudest description of what constituted melancholia, or mental defectiveness, or what not, and without our having any understanding about the significance of their acts or how to deal with them. Violence was met by violence, hyperactivity was met by restraint, wakefulness was dealt with by hypnotics; and that constituted in principle the whole story except for the fact that here and there was the intuitive individual who just naturally understood his patients, knew what to expect and how to get the best results in handling them. These intuitive people, as I have already indicated, were not infrequently attendants, and while their extraordinary capacity was recognized and their services were appreciated they were not understood.

Perhaps I can best give some idea of the revolutionary change that occurred by saying that in the nineteenth century mind was considered as an epiphenomenon, something added to the organism. Just when it was added or how it was added were questions that not only were not answered but were not often asked; it was just the way in which one thought about the mind as a super-imposed structure of some sort. It was thought of as a static affair, whereas the changed viewpoint thought of it as a process not static but dynamic, not structural but functional.

It was but the natural evolution of the theory of evolution itself that mind should necessarily have to come to be considered in this way. It had long been realized that somehow the gap between the inorganic and the organic would have to be filled up, that life did not just happen on the earth but that it came to pass as a result of certain processes which in their beginnings took place within the framework of the inorganic. While no one has bridged this gap as yet, it is beginning to be more and more possible to think about it as being bridged because of the added information that science is furnishing every day as to the nature of the various processes that are going on in the universe. However that may be, the same problem in kind confronts the origin of mind, if one wants to stick to the old idea of mind as a superstructure. There must at some time have come into existence mind, and there must have been some time before this when there was no such thing. Personally I have discarded this view for one which perhaps I could not defend very successfully against a competent opponent but which seems to me to offer definite advantages. Mind from my point of view is merely one aspect of the functioning of the organism, namely, the functioning of the organism-as-a-whole. As I repeatedly illustrate, the minute we begin to say of a man that he is doing this, that or the other thing, we are necessarily committed to the use of language that describes his conduct in psychological terms. The whole scheme of evolution, therefore, commits us to the assumption that what is happening in nature can not be expressed by a static terminology but can only be understood as something that is going on continuously, or, as I have said above, something that is in process.

It will be seen from the above that what has happened since the nineteenth century is that man is being really assimilated to the rest of the cosmos, that he is accepting himself as having not only evolved from the lower animals but he is even accepting the life within him as having originally come from the inorganic world and his mind as one aspect of that expression of his living organism which has had a similar origin. Every movement in the way of belief has been away from the old idea that man was especially created, that he was the special object of God's solicitude, and that the earth and the rest of the universe were made on purpose for him. This view and the one that is now coming into existence are diametrically opposed. The grandeur of man is not in his isolation but in his allegiance to the rest of the cosmos. The old idea was essentially additive in nature. Not only was mind added somewhere along the way but the nervous system was made up of a multiplication of reflex arcs, one added to another, not only increasing the number but the complexities and the possibilities of reaction. The body was composed of cells, cells added to one another, etc., and in the old academic psychology we have the same thing. We have functions of the mind apparently independent of each other but added together in making up the total picture. This additive way of thinking has given place to the dynamic and the functional ways of thinking, and so far as these relate to the mind in particular I have expressed myself elsewhere* as follows:

" The old structural academic psychology assumed that on the psychological side the finished product, the idea for example, could be traced back to its elemental constituents, which in this instance were sensations. The sensation was the unit of psychic structure and the psychic state at any particular moment was a mosaic of such sensations, very much as one might conceive a bit of matter to be a mosaic of molecules. Similarly the nervous system was constructed of units. In this case the unit was the reflex, and the complicated processes of the higher centers were but mathematical summaries of reflex arcs. During the present century, however, these views have been slowly changing. The study of child psychology, for example, has demonstrated that the child does not acquire first a series of discrete sensations and then put them together so as to form perceptions, etc., so that these perceptions are nothing more nor less than the sum of the sensations which compose them. This limiting mechanistic hypothesis has been headed for the discard for some time and is now definitely in the waste-basket. The child's first experiences are not of such a nature. The first experiences are comparable, using a biological analogy, to the protoplasm which is the basic substance of life. The first experiences of the child are already perceptions, perceptions with respect to which it attempts to relate itself. The difference between these perceptions, as the difference between protoplasm and the higher forms of life, is a difference in differentiation. The specific and the concrete are not amalgamated to make the complex, but out of a relatively homogeneous background these concrete constructs differentiate and emerge; so that development and evolution proceed by a process of differentiation and emergence and it becomes evident that the whole is not expressed in the sum of its parts but the whole is more than the sum of its parts, for by the organization of the parts and their relation to each other something enters the situation which is possessed by none of those parts separately."

From this point of view what we see in evolutional development is the process of differentiation rather than of addition.

This changed viewpoint is nothing more nor less than a complete about-face from the viewpoint of the nineteenth century. Mind is no longer considered as an isolated phenomenon in the universe but is considered as related to the universe in the same way that everything else is related, as an expression, the culminating expression, of the processes which have been going on in this universe from the

---

* Outlines of Psychiatry. Nervous and Mental Disease Monograph Series No. 1, 13th Edition, p. 7.

beginning of time. Therefore man becomes a part of the cosmos in a way in which he never was before. It is easy to see how such a complete change of front in considering man's place in nature should alter the way in which we look at the specific problems which he presents. For example, it is much more compatible with this point of view that psychological phenomena should be considered from the deterministic standpoint. The concept of free will will have to be at least very much modified even if actual determinism is not fully accepted. The acceptance, however, of the deterministic attitude is one of the aspects of the development in psychology in the present century, and, like so many other things that can not be definitely defined or proved, its utility can be disclosed in the results which it produces; for the investigation of mental phenomena on the theory that they are not merely haphazard occurrences but are determined by what went before, just as the physical events of the universe are bound up in their antecedents, has resulted in an enormous enlargement of the understanding of what happens in the realm of the psychic. So that from this point of view, at least, determinism has thoroughly justified itself. The question from a philosophical point of view is somewhat different and does not interest us here.

Another concept which was also brought into the picture by way of the psychoanalytic movement, and which has been quite as significant in the results which have flown from it as that of determinism, is the concept of the unconscious. As we look back upon the last century we can understand how impossible it was for either man or his mind to be adequately understood in relation to the universe so long as mind was understood solely in terms of consciousness; but when the psyche, as it does now, came to include not only consciousness but a vast number of additional phenomena, then for the first time it was possible to understand the significance of mind and its meaning, which is tantamount to saying that for the first time it was possible to begin to understand man himself. To revert to an analogy used by Professor G. Stanley Hall, previous to the acceptance of the concept of the unconscious we were in the same position in undertaking to explain man's motives as we would have been had we attempted to explain the movement of an iceberg when we could see that the iceberg was moving in a direction exactly opposite to the prevailing wind. As long as we limited our observation to the visible portion of the iceberg and took into consideration only the wind, the movement of the iceberg contrary to the direction of the wind would forever remain inexplicable; but when we come to realize that nine-tenths of the iceberg was submerged and that this submerged portion was subject to ocean currents and that these currents were moving in a direction the opposite of the wind, then we could understand how the iceberg as we saw it above the surface of the sea could be moved contrary to the wind. And so long as we knew nothing about the unconscious we knew nothing about those deeper currents in man's psyche that motivated his conduct. So long as we saw only his actual conduct and were restricted to the field of consciousness for its explanation we could never understand him. The concept of the unconscious enabled us to realize that these motives came from beneath—using a spatial analogy—the field of consciousness, and served for the first time to enable us to explain things which before had been inexplicable.

It is worth while to pause for a moment and try to comprehend the enormous difference that separates the concept of mind of the nineteenth century from that of the present day. Forty years ago when I started my study of psychiatry the mind was a series of phenomena which were little known, elaborately described and confined entirely to the field of consciousness. Mental phenomena belonged primarily to human beings although the lower animals were generally accredited with simple psychological types of reaction, but no one ever thought of attributing psychological phenomena to animals lower in the scale than the mammals or higher vertebrates, and certainly no one ever thought of attributing such phemonema to plants. Mind in accordance with the general theory of those days was an additive phenomenon. It had been added somewhere along the path of evolution. Now in the twentieth century we see an exceedingly different sort of picture. We see that inasmuch as life itself must have come over the bridge that separates the inorganic from the organic that the laws that govern life can not be essentially different in their broad expressions from those that govern in the inorganic world. We are prepared, for example, to see action and reaction, equal and in opposite directions, expressed in both fields. If this concept is accepted, then it must also be accepted that psychological phenomena are not something that have been added as it was formerly supposed that one reflex had been added to another, but that they are only certain aspects of life reactions and therefore wherever we find life we will find psychological types of reaction as well as other types. Here again we are confronted by the necessity if we make this first assumption of following it by the assumption that the laws of the psyche are not different from the laws of the rest of the cosmos, because if life has come over the bridge from the inorganic to the organic the possibility of psychological types of manifestation has also. The psyche, as it seems to me, is an environmental inclusion, an easy enough conception when one is thinking of the taking in and making a part of one's self of cultural standards but perhaps not quite so easy to understand in its larger biological significance.

We always in the past thought of the mind as receptive to the various experiences from the outside world that came by way of the five special senses. We know now that this is altogether too simplistic an idea of the processes of reception even, and that instead of there being five senses there are over twenty and that these include such sensations as result in response to gravity and which are outside of the field of consciousness. But we are thinking in this twentieth century also of the projected interests of the individual. We see the great cultural institutions, religion, law, morals, economics, etc., as modifications of the environment produced by the individual to meet his needs. They are the projected and evolved interests of the individual. So from this point of view the mind becomes literally a microcosm, that is, a small cosmos, as it includes all of the universe of which man is cognizant. Not only by a process of reception through sense organs does it know this cosmos but by a process of projected interests, which interests themselves evolve, does it modify and change that cosmos to his own purposes. In this way we see that the concept of the individual and the environment are not mutually exclusive. Here again we are dealing only with two aspects of phenomena which include them both, a conclusion which is inevitable if life has come up from the inorganic, as we must accept that it has. It is but an outgrowth of the conditions of the environment and therefore expresses them in its response to the same laws. Mind, therefore, instead of being an epiphenomenon which is the characteristic of only a few animals, has become all-pervading, takes in and gives out throughout every portion of the known universe—not a pan-psychism in the sense that mind as a substance is in all these parts of the universe, but in the sense that man can only contact with the universe by means of his mind. He can only modify the universe as a result of his mental processes and therefore everything mental concentrates in him, and that includes his perceptions and his reactions thereto.

# CHAPTER XV

## MEDICAL PSYCHOLOGY

Of very great importance in the expansion of the psychiatric viewpoint was the development, as I have already indicated, of a psychology which differed very essentially from the old academic type which had held the stage for so long. Academic psychology at the end of the nineteenth and the beginning of the twentieth century was still confined to a description of the processes as they could be discerned within the field of consciousness plus those additions which had come from applying the laboratory methods of the Wundtian school. It was a mixture of description at the conscious level with still some attachments to its old philosophical moorings plus an addition of neural physiology which latter permitted the introduction of exact methods of measurement. The new psychology which grew up as a result of the direct study of the mentally ill and which was stimulated and fostered largely by the psychoanalytic school originally in its studies of the neuroses was very different in type. It was not primarily interested in the field of consciousness but rather in the field of the unconscious. It was not primarily interested in the intellectual field but rather in the field of the emotions. It dealt with man not as a text-book construct, but as a living, feeling, desiring organism being driven in certain directions by instinctual tendencies and reacting to his environment in accordance with his personality pattern, on the one hand, and the nature and quality of the environment, on the other. The psychological aspects of human behavior had come to be thought of as only one aspect from which the individual might be viewed; and just as the amoeba structurally might be thought of as the most primitive expression of what millions of years later became the enormously complicated structural system of man, so the amoeba in action might be thought of as being the most primitive expression of what later became man's psyche.

If these fundamental considerations are correct then it follows naturally that all disease has its psychic components and that nineteenth century medicine, which was essentially a development of medicine along somatic lines, failed because of its lack of appreciation of this fact to present a complete picture of a disease process.

Every living creature, from our point of view then, has not only somatic but psychic aspects. Disease, therefore, not only may have psychogenic factors but must necessarily have psychological components. To illustrate this point of view, which is of the utmost significance for medicine in general and which is an outgrowth of the development of psychiatry, I will quote at some length what I have said elsewere, as follows :*

"As has already been intimated, the medicine of the past has developed preponderantly along somatic lines and in the direction of specialization, so that highly trained men have been functioning only too often as technicians interested in diseases and organs rather than in sick individuals. Psychiatry in its recent developments has been the only medical specialty that because of its nature was called upon to deal with the whole individual in any real sense. While other medical specialists gave lip service to the idea of treating the sick person rather than the disease, psychiatry really was forced more nearly to acting upon this principle than any other specialty; and now it has come about as a result of psychiatric investigations, psychiatric thought and the psychiatric point of view, that the individual has come to be vastly more important than any of his diseases or his organs. In fact the concept that considers the organism as a whole, and the necessary correlate thereto, that there is a psychological factor in every illness, bids fair to cause a revolution in medical thinking that will be of as great significance and as radical in its results as the revolution that has recently come about in the thinking of the physicists and the astronomers.

" To have launched such concepts as thinking by the phantasy method, the hypothesis of the unconscious, the theory of determinism in the psychic sphere, and to have come to a realization of the factual significance of ideas as well as the impossibility of determining the nature of the reality back of them, to appreciate the significance of the emotional cross-currents of a personality and the inability of the individual to face his instinctive tendencies, to have done away with such misconceptions as are based upon the body-mind dilemma and to have come to a realization that psychology is a biological science and to an understanding that pathological processes are only different from so-called normal process in degree and emphasis and that disorder and disease in the mental sphere are experiments of Nature from which the observer can learn about the normal, healthy functions of the mind,—to have launched such a series of concepts as this and many others into the field of mental medicine is as radical a thing in the field of science as were the contributions of

* Medical Psychology. Nervous and Mental Disease Monograph Series No. 54, p. 133.

Copernicus, of Newton and of Pasteur; while to be able to study and identify mental processes, to bring them within the operation of formulated laws, to realize that in this sphere the phenomena of emergent evolution are visible, and to begin to believe that the same laws govern in the sphere of the mind as do in the sphere of the body and that these laws are again the same as operate in the inorganic environment because the living being together with his psychological mechanisms is a stamped-in environmental inclusion, is to think in terms which are bound to radically modify all of our attitudes towards our patients either from the viewpoint of considering the whys and wherefores or from the viewpoint of attempting to formulate a system of therapy. Our concept of the nature of the world that we live in inevitably reflects itself in our conduct in relation to that world.

" Let us close by just mentioning a few of the significant conclusions and important implications of what has gone before, and in doing so remember that in trying to push forward into the unknown we must have the courage to speculate and to believe with Huxley that: ' He that does not go beyond the facts will seldom get as far as the facts.' In the first place, if for every state of the soma there is a corresponding state of the psyche, if the mind never exists at any moment without being at the same time psychologically active, we get a slant upon therapeutics which while it is not new and has repeatedly been referred to is still not by any means sufficiently borne in mind. In fact to all intents and purposes it is entirely ignored. The slant I refer to is to the effect that every method of treatment is at the same time a form of psychotherapy. No matter whether the physician administers a drug, prescribes a dietetic or hygienic regime or performs a surgical operation, the influence of these measures upon the patient's psyche should never be lost sight of. Especially is it obvious in chronic diseases. There are certain diseases like epilepsy where almost everything known to medicine has been reported as effecting a cure. Under such circumstances naturally none of the things that have been reported have effected the cure but if there has been a cure or an amelioration the chances are that it has been produced by the influence of the therapy upon the mind of the patient, in other words by means of something that was common to all of the various therapies employed. The whole realm of chronic disease becomes immediately of different significance. When the microscope, the test tube, and the X-ray have failed, it is certainly time to interrogate the mind. There is really no excuse for further going on with the usual methods of investigation of diseases which have failed to yield their secrets for generations without at least at the same time trying to find out whether there may not be adequate psychogenic factors involved. For the implication of all that has been said before is that the foundations of the personality are laid down in early life and if they are laid down askew, as it were, then does the individual grow up with a distorted personality, which distorted personality in its influence upon the body, constantly year in and year out bending the body as its tool to satisfy its ends and bring its wishes to pass, ultimately produces the phenomena of some of the chronic illnesses which we know only too well.

"Another significant fact which issues from the structure that the previous pages have built up and from what I have just said about distorted personalities is that the mental hospital is the place above all others which has been neglected in the study of medicine.    It has been recognized for a long time that the autopsy room was a most valuable adjunct in correcting errors of diagnosis and in increasing information about disease and helping to teach, because there finally the physician was brought face to face with the facts whereas up to that time he had merely been inferring them.    This is all true, but the same thing applies, and perhaps more emphatically, to the mental hospital.    The great number of patients who arrive there suffering with mental disease have been getting sick for years.    Some of them have been getting sick for twenty or thirty or forty years, and their illness is an end result of this twisted personality that we have been discussing.    In the course of their illness they have been through the hands of innumerable doctors, sometimes as many as forty or fifty, and these various physicians have done everything conceivable to these patients in the line of therapy.    Quite frequently they have at one or another time gotten into the hands of the surgeon and they may come to the hospital after having had numerous major operations and several of their organs enucleated. The mental hospital is the place of last resort.    When the patients have exhausted the resources of the family practitioner, and incidentally their own financial resources, then they come to the mental hospital and then is the time to study in longitudinal section their life histories, and the part that medicine has played therein.    Adequate studies of this sort would be of enormous significance to the future progress of therapeutics.    It would not be necessary to wait until the patient got to the dead-house in order to find out some very significant facts.

"If one surveys the field of psychiatry as it has broadened out during the past quarter century, as it has attempted the solution of questions not only in mental medicine and in preventive medicine but in criminology, industry, education, child rearing, and innumerable other things, one must realize that the field of psychiatry as thus exploited by these ambitious proponents is no less than the problem of civilization itself; and when one discusses what constitutes an adequate curriculum in the medical schools so that the student coming out therefrom may have a grasp of this subject it is quite natural to feel overwhelmed and impotent in the face of the immensity of the problem and the short period of time that the medical school has to give it. This would be all true if the facts that had to be learned were discrete and disconnected. It would be like learning the facts of the physical universe before the days of Newton, when the fall of a pebble or an apple was one phenomenon, the tides of the ocean another, the orderly revolution of the planets in their spheres still another, and so on throughout an infinity of natural phenomena discrete and disconnected. Then came the law of gravity, and all of these apparently disconnected manifestations dropped into the mold of a single formula, and the result can only be described as an amazing simplification of what up to that time had been an equally amazing complexity. We have a perfect right if our surmises in the previous pages have been correct to expect the same sort of thing to happen in the sphere of mental phenomena. In fact it is so happening. We know, for example, that love and affection do not exist in 100 per cent concentration, that all the happenings in the mental sphere in the field of the emotions or feelings are ambivalent, that wherever we find love and affection we find it diluted with some degree of aggressiveness. And so we are prepared by knowing that general principle for a host of phenomena. Take, for example, the disturbances that occur in the course of impregnation, pregnancy and parturition. Take the young woman who is afraid of becoming pregnant, who after she becomes pregnant is afraid of the risks incident to parturition, who during the early days of her pregnancy is uncomfortable and later on develops nausea and vomiting, who feels ashamed of the change in her appearance and retires from contact with other people and who finally has a prolonged, painful and difficult labor and subsequently is unable for any length of time to nurse her child because she has not sufficient milk, etc., etc. Is it not possible to explain all these phenomena simply rather than to seek in the disturbances of metabolism and organ function and diet and general health and constitution and predisposition, and all the other places that are familiar to us, for causes? If none of these disclose any information that is satisfactory and we interrogate the Unconscious of this young woman, the Unconscious might tell us something like the following, which will be significant if we remember that the Unconscious is guided solely by the pleasure principle. So the Unconscious might inform us that it had arranged itself a very nice time, it had made all the preparations for a trip around the world and a thousand and one details had been filled in in imagination, all of which would be entrancingly interesting, delightful and satisfying. Then along comes this pregnancy. The hostess of the Unconscious, the body, gets into this difficulty, a difficulty which she had attempted to avoid but which nevertheless accidentally occurred, and now the whole picture is changed. The trip around the world will have to be given up. Not only that, here is a period of several months during most of which none of the usual satisfactions to which she has been accustomed can be indulged, and beyond that years and years of responsibility. Is it not easy to see how the advent of a pregnancy is resented by this pleasure-seeking Unconscious, how the new creature that is coming into being instead of being looked forward to with expectation and love and impatience, etc., is looked forward to as a little brat and that all manner of dire thoughts are directed against it even to the extent of wishing it would die or desiring to get rid of it at all costs? And when we find women who actually respond to such impulses and do kill their children, can we not see that we are merely at one extreme of a situation which in more diluted form affects everyone who is faced by a new responsibility, and so are we not justified in the opinion that psychological laws will evolve that are as significant and simplifying in their results as we are accustomed to seeing in the physical world? In addition to this we see with what force constructive factors, even when inadequate, manifest themselves in a personality such as that described. Such a person would most undoubtedly be of infantile make-up and inadequately developed on the emotional side for the responsibilities of parenthood, and yet the creative urge is so great that its partial repression or attempted repression along the lines indicated produces an enormous amount of compensatory suffering as a result of her continual illness. At the psychological level there would probably lie back of such a picture intense feelings of guilt and an equally intense need for punishment. Nature, so to speak, makes every effort to produce adults capable of the great responsibilities of life. In the case cited the illness was the indication of the degree of failure in this process.

"Then there is a word of caution which issues after having considered all the various things that have come up for discussion in the preceding pages. It has been plainly set forth that in the realm of mental disorder we are dealing primarily with drives, tendencies, desires which are of emotional nature fundamentally rather than of intellectual or rational significance. In other words, the psychology of mental disorders from this point of view is a psychology of the irrational as opposed to the rational. I mention this here because it is a common fault of almost everyone to attempt to appeal to the mentally disordered individual on rational grounds. How often has it not happened that the physician has attempted to dislodge a delusion or a fear by resort to reason and logic, and how often has this effort failed, because it must fail in the majority of instances? The language of the emotions is not the language of reason. And so we are dealing in this sphere with the irrational components of mind, and the various situations which are created by them must be finessed rather than approached head on by an appeal to cold facts.

Herein lies the contribution which has recently been made in the field of psychotherapy.

"Another aspect of the therapy of mental illnesses lies along the same line. Probably because of our tremendous success in recent generations, particularly in the last century, in the realm of science, we have come to have what is perhaps an exaggerated opinion of the value of the intellect. Perhaps it would be better to turn it about and say that we have neglected to appreciate the emotional side of life. There was in the old days, some two thousand or so years ago, a problem which was set for the mathematician to solve. The problem was that of the tortoise and the athlete, and it was demonstrated in this problem that no matter how he tried the swift-running athlete could never pass the tortoise; and for all these years great scientific intellects have struggled with this problem, but life did not have to struggle with it. No matter how deeply these scientific intellects became involved in their fruitless reasonings no one, however simple in mind, for a moment doubted that the athlete could pass the tortoise and life held no example to the contrary.

" Someone has said that we do not live but ' are lived,' and if we are lived it is by these old instinctive tendencies that have been stamped into our make-up for millions of years. Psychotherapy does not undertake to tell people what they ought to do. No one is wise enough to do that, and if the physician undertook it he would only succeed in giving his patient his own personal formula. What psychotherapy does attempt to do, however, is to release the individual from the domination of regressive tendencies and infantile fixations. When this is done the energy so released will fly to creative purposes of its own accord. I mention this only because it is one of the aspects of psychotherapy which has been sorely misunderstood.

" Many another thing might be brought up in this summary to show how the point of view developed in the preceding pages must necessarily modify not only our way of thinking but our way of doing. I have already referred particularly to the contributions of Copernicus, of Darwin and of Freud, and have indicated that the resistances to these contributions were the results of wounding man's narcissism. I suspect that an adequate grasp of the real place that man holds in nature,* his relation to his environment and to other human organisms along the lines that I have built up in this book, involves an additional wound to man's narcissism, and that he will not take kindly to a scientific approach to an understanding of himself which requires as a pre-condition the renunciation of all of the childish tendencies and childish securities. But the facts of science as they slowly emerge from the unknown and become susceptible of proof have to be accepted and are unyielding. The following quotations

* See my Meaning of Disease, published by Williams and Wilkins.

from the English astronomer Jeans* will give some idea of where
man stands in the cosmos as the cosmos is conceived by the
modern astronomer: 'A few stars are known which are hardly
bigger than the earth, but the majority are so large that hundreds
of thousands of earths could be packed inside each and leave
room to spare; here and there we come upon a giant star large
enough to contain millions of millions of earths. And the total
number of stars in the universe is probably something like the
total number of grains of sand on all the seashores of the world.
Such is the littleness of our home in space when measured up
against the total substance of the universe.' . . . 'Is this,
then, all that life amounts to? To stumble, almost by mistake,
into a universe which was clearly not designed for life, and
which, to all appearances, is either totally indifferent or definitely
hostile to it, to stay clinging onto a fragment of a grain of sand
until we are frozen off, to strut our tiny hour on our tiny stage
with the knowledge that our aspirations are all doomed to final
frustration, and that our achievements must perish with our race,
leaving the universe as though we had never been?'

"These quotations are by no means intended to make man
take life less seriously or feel that nothing is worth while or
assume a fatalistic attitude of doing nothing about anything, for
after all this is the only life that we have to live, it is our life and
it is ours to make the best of as best we can. But if man's
narcissism is going to be wounded I can conceive of no more
dangerous weapon than the two paragraphs just quoted and perhaps it would have been well to have started this book with these
paragraphs rather than to have ended it with them, for surely the
absence of a narcissistic overemphasis is a splendid preparation
for a knowledge of one's self.

"The intellectual growth of man may be sketched, beginning
with his disillusionment as the result of doing away with his
simplistic conceptions of the universe in the scheme of which he
regarded himself as the special object of creation and everything
else subordinate to him. This was followed by the further disillusionment brought to fruition by the theory of evolution, and a
still further wound to his narcissism was suffered on the advent
of psychoanalysis. Man reacted to each of these serious affronts
to his egotism by adequate compensations which resulted, respec-
tively, in his mastering by means of his intellect the physical
universe, the field of biology and the facts of psychology. Now
in these later days when the X-ray and radium and the advances
of physics generally have destroyed the nineteenth century concept
of matter upon which man had rested for so long as a firm
foundation of safety he feels the last bit of assurance from
sources outside of himself slipping away, and he is not only being

* Jeans, Sir James: The Mysterious Universe. The Macmillan Co., New
York, 1930.

relentlessly pushed by the increasing force of the facts of science to feel that his only salvation must rest in his ability to stand upon his own feet but he is now being allied and identified with the inanimate aspects of Nature as he was before with his fellows and with all life. We have to acknowledge that the laws of science that control within the realm of his most secret places take away the last vestige of his individuality as he feels it, but on the other hand if the analogy with the other instances given holds in this instance they must of necessity set loose compensatory mechanisms and thus start in operation creative impulses at another level of activity which will result in still further depriving him of the crutches of illusion and forcing him into ever more effective ways of facing and dealing with reality."

This, in brief, is the sort of psychology which has grown up, mostly during the present century, as a result of the study by the physician of his individual patients and their difficulties. It will be seen that it has nothing of the characteristics of the old academic psychologies of the universities and owes little or nothing to them for what it has accomplished. It is a psychology, however, which not only has been formulated as a result of treating effectively and intelligently sick individuals but it has grown up under the conditions of twentieth century scientific development and it reflects the new concepts, the new ways of thinking which have been developed by man's efforts at a more adequate understanding of his cosmos and as a result of his conviction that the concepts and the ways of thinking of the last century must needs be abandoned because they have served their purpose and they have nothing further to contribute.

Of course it must be understood that this type of psychology is not accepted by everyone today, not even by the physicians, not even by the psychiatrists. It is, in my opinion, the sort of psychology, however, which is forcing its way to recognition and which in essence represents the ways of thinking and the concepts which will rule in this sphere for some time to come. Psychiatry and medicine in adopting such a psychology has to leave behind its old-fashioned static formulations, has to leave behind such limiting and today useless concepts as "insanity," disease, and the like, and such ambivalent opposites as body-mind, heredity-environment, and a host of other oppositions of this sort. The new psychology is unifying in its tendencies and dynamic in its principles. Body and mind are merely different aspects of the organism, different ways of envisaging it for different purposes. Heredity and environment can not be separated. They again are only different aspects of the phenomena which may be utilized separately for certain purposes but which can not exist apart. The whole story of life from the very beginning negates any such possibility.

Perhaps of all the scientific disciplines that deal with human individuals criminology retains at the present moment the greatest number of these hangovers from old ways of thinking in the nature of static concepts which are seriously interfering with this branch of learning, such concepts as crime and criminals, the ideas which are behind such words as " punishment," and such highly metaphysical concepts as responsibility, and " insanity " as being tantamount to irresponsibility. All such ideas as these must be cast aside before any clear thinking in accordance with the tendencies of modern science will be possible; but if we read the literature of the day with an open mind we find that all these highly desirable changes are in fact taking place. They are not taking place consciously, the change is not being intentionally directed; but the new problems that arise and the new methods that have to be invented for their solution, and the coming together in these various problems of several branches of science, and the continued inadequacy of the old concepts and the old methods, are gradually bringing to pass changes in the directions I have indicated, all of which means that it is reasonable to expect that progress along all of these lines of endeavor will take place rapidly from now on.

# CHAPTER XVI

## HOSPITAL ADMINISTRATION

In the preceding pages I have tried to indicate the way in which psychiatry developed from the position it occupied forty years ago, how it became of increasing significance and importance medically, socially, legally and scientifically, how the practice of psychiatry expanded until it broke down the barrier of the asylum walls and entered into many extra-mural activities, and how its development along all lines not only widened the horizon of this medical specialty but brought it into line with changing and developing thought as we find it expressed in the present century in all branches of learning. Psychiatry has not only helped to define man's place in nature and to make that place a much more dignified one and one of very much enlarged significance, but psychiatry has found a place for itself which is harmoniously related not only to the other medical specialties but to the whole body of scientific thought.

If the reader up to this point has appreciated the part that the hospital, particularly the state hospital, has played in the evolution of psychiatry and psychiatric thought, he will be prepared to understand that the hospital had to respond to all these wide-reaching changes that I have just mentioned. The old asylum of the middle of the nineteenth century was very little better than a hotel where the patients were the guests. The superintendent, a kindly man, was busy with its management, assisted by a steward who looked after the feeding of the patients, and the principal business operations, generally with the assistance of a bookkeeper. The superintendent looked after the general health of the place, usually with the assistance of two or three doctors as there were usually five hundred to a thousand patients and these doctors attended to the sick in a routine sort of manner which did not require much of them in the way of diagnosis or therapy. The superintendent's principal reliance was upon occupational therapy, and occupational therapy in those days meant working on the farm. I do not intend by any means to underrate the superintendent of this period, as what I have said in previous chapters indicates; but after all, his job was a relatively simple one, from the medical point of view, in comparison with what it has now become. The armamentarium of medicine in general, and of psychiatry in particular, has enormously increased, and it has become one of the functions of the hospital to bring all these various diagnostic and therapeutic agencies which have been developed through the years to the service of the patient in a large hospital. This alone required considerable modification of administrative plan and procedure. In addition to this the country as a whole has grown, population has increased, the number of patients in the state hospital has mounted, the expense of running these institutions has become a very material portion of the state budget, and social, legal and economic complications have entered the picture and made the whole hospital situation a much more difficult and intricate affair than it used to be. Added to this was the old-time superstition that doctors never made good administrators, and the old-time inertia that prevented any administrative scheme from undergoing developmental changes. Where the first idea came from I have never known, except that as a rule doctors were not administrators. They were busy practising their profession, and sometimes doing so without adequately looking after what other people seemed to think were their own interests, namely, their money affairs. I have personally, however, known numbers of doctors who made outstanding administrators, and I have always felt that this idea that they were constitutionally unequal to the task of administration was founded upon a myth, in the first instance, and that its continued existence was dependent upon wishful thinking of the various individuals and groups who wanted to absorb the administrative jobs that otherwise the doctors would naturally be expected to do. However, I feel that the last forty years have demonstrated over and over again that the running of a hospital, no matter how complicated it may become, how much it may grow, is the job of a physician, and that just as soon as one is willing to concede to the physician the possibility that he may do this kind of job it will be found quite as easy to obtain one that is competent as it is to obtain one trained in any other way. Everything about a hospital, directly or indirectly, has medical significance, medical implications; and peculiarly this is true of the hospital for mental disease, for these institutions are built not only to take in the acutely ill but to keep those who can not get well and make as satisfactory adjustments as possible for them the rest of their lives. Under these circumstances the management of the environment of the mentally ill is a function that no one should have the last word about except the psychiatrist.

All sorts of schemes have been devised for running hospitals other than having a medical superintendent to do it, but in my opinion none of them have succeeded.  Even though some of them have apparently succeeded financially and apparently succeeded over a certain period of time, there is one feature of the situation which has always been overlooked.  A hospital is like a miniature society.  It develops its cultural ideals in the same way and it is exceedingly important that these cultural ideals that are accumulated through the years should have come from the right fountain-heads, that they should have been medically conceived in the first instance, and that they should in their turn help to build up enduring traditions which have as their objective the welfare of the patient and which are based upon that profound understanding of the patient which no one but the physician, so far as I know, can be expected to have.  Paid executives, political appointees, can never possibly take the place of the representative of the profession which is consecrated to the patient; and if the individual in that profession be himself a better-than-ordinary man, then the hospital is doubly blessed.  I have seen these various experiments of lay control tried here and there and I am sure they fail in these more significant ways that I have mentioned, and that they can never be expected to succeed because of their natural, inherent defects along these lines.

With the growth of medicine, particularly along the lines of specialization, with the growing recognition that the patients in the great state hospitals were entitled to the relief that the medical sciences could extend to them freely if they were not in such institutions, it became necessary to devise ways for having the specialist see the patient in the hospital.  This was a comparatively easy procedure and it was negotiated by having regular dispensary days so that the ophthalmologist, the laryngologist, the dentist, etc., came to the hospital, say for a half day each week.  These were matters of detail which were not difficult to adjust.

Perhaps one of the most important things that has happened in the whole field of hospital administration in the last forty years has been the growing recognition that hospital administration itself is a medical specialty.  The great American Hospital Association has undertaken to provide educational opportunities for those who wish to go into this profession and has set up minimum standards of requirements for those who enter its ranks.  To be sure, up to the present moment these opportunities and these standards referred particularly to the superintendents of general hospitals rather than to superintendents of hospitals for mental disease, but the movement is a movement in the right direction without doubt. One of the fundamental principles that lies at the basis of this entire movement, to my way of thinking, is that hospital administration is as much a matter of research as any other medical specialty, and that as the hospitals in this country are becoming increasingly complex and growing rapidly in size this research field becomes progressively more and more important, because there are no precedents upon which to base the development of the administrative mechanisms that must be brought to bear upon the situation.

In the old days there was a period when it was believed that no hospital for mental diseases ought to have over 500 beds. Despite this accepted maximum standard of size, the hospitals grew beyond this and finally the maximum was advanced to 1,000 beds. Nevertheless the hospitals continued to grow and the maximum was again raised to 1,500 beds. Since then I am not aware that anyone has had the temerity to say how large a hospital ought to be. As a matter of fact the hospitals are continuing to grow. Saint Elizabeths Hospital, for example, now has 5,000 beds, and the new Pilgrim Hospital in New York is designed to have ultimately 10,000 beds. The size of the hospital is dictated by a great many factors, not the least of which is the delay of legislatures in providing beds as fast as they are needed and in creating new institutions. It is quite true that 500, 1,000 or 1,500 beds is a proper maximum to place upon the size of an institution for mental diseases provided there is no change in the administrative methods. No hospital of 5,000 beds can possibly be run in accordance with the administrative standards of a hospital of 500 to 1,000 beds, which means that as a hospital grows the administrative scheme must keep up with the procession and be varied to take care of the added problems and the increased complexities that arise along the way. At Saint Elizabeths, for example, I should say there have been during my incumbency some three pretty complete readjustments of the whole administrative scheme; and I might almost say that as a measure for such readjustments it could be roughly stated that every time a hospital grows sufficiently to need an addition to the power house, new boilers and electric generators, it will be necessary to remodel the administrative scheme.

One other thing about hospital administration that occurs to me as fairly fundamental is that centralization and decentralization are its systole and diastole. As a hospital grows up to a certain size there is a tendency to more and more concentrate the authority at a single point, let us say the administrative building; but when the hospital gets beyond this certain size, when its individual units get to be say the size of a hospital of a generation ago, 1,000 or 1,500 beds, then it becomes desirable that these units be decentralized, administered as separate institutions, and that the centralized authority in the administration building should be rearranged. Chiefs of service then have the same qualifications, let us say, that superintendents had in the old days, and the superintendent of the whole institution then becomes by analogy the state hospital commission.

I wish in the few words of this chapter to convey the thought that the advances along the various lines that psychiatry has made, particularly in the more strictly medical fields, have necessarily had their influence upon the administrative lay-out of the big hospitals, and that in order that these advances may continue and accomplish their purposes adequately it is essential that this administrative scheme should grow correspondingly to meet the necessities which they create. This is what is happening, and I have indicated very briefly how it is happening. It is by no means an unimportant part of the problem because even with the development of extra-mural psychiatry there remain these hundreds of thousands of patients that have to be cared for in these big institutions, and the economic, the legal, the social and the administrative aspects of these problems have to be taken into consideration as well as the strictly medical aspects. I can remember in the old days that the young physician, the same type of individual that I have described previously as having turned up his nose at the hospital superintendent, used to say that he could not waste his time in administrative matters. His business was the practice of medicine and it was beneath his dignity to look into such homely concerns as the housekeeping of the institution, the hiring of chambermaids, or even the garnering of the harvest, the cutting of the crops, the taking care of the cows, looking after the milk supply, whereas when it came to the matter of laying water pipes, and, more terrible than all else, sewer pipes, why these things were just beneath contempt and no really self-respecting psychiatrist would ever lend himself to such purposes. Of course these are but the vaporings of adolescent incapacities, the childish egotisms that compensate for inadequacies and lack of wisdom. The real situation, of course, is that the superintendent maintains the great physical establishment where all manner of medical and scientific work may be conducted. How much scientific work could possibly go on if the power plant shut down and there was no light and no heat in winter and no water in summer, or if the physical integrity of the plant were permitted to get into such shape that the roofs were not safe, etc., etc.? These may be homely tasks but they are exceedingly important. They are as important to the hospital as the heart is important to the individual. All these things must work, and so the superintendent who maintains this kind of establishment is doing infinitely more than he could ever do himself in his individual capacity by treating patients. He is giving perhaps fifty scientifically trained men opportunities to practice their specialty and to discover new scientific truths. Very few can have greater opportunities than the hospital superintendent for worthwhile influence in their lives, even though the opportunity in this instance is frequently vicariously availed of. The superintendent certainly is doing a much more important job, probably, than any one of his assistants, and a very much more important job than he could possibly do by himself unless he happened to be a genius. So that the modern hospital with its modern administrative scheme represents a highly specialized development where psychiatry is best studied, and not only psychiatry alone but all the diseases and particularly the chronic ones that affect human beings, for here patients come to spend the rest of their days. They live for twenty, thirty, forty years and sometimes more. One gets unexampled opportunities to study the longitudinal section of their life histories and to follow it by the pathological findings after the end has come. These great hospitals are only beginning to be appreciated for what they really are, outstanding opportunities for medical research.

To return to the matter of the size of a hospital. I have indicated that in the past several limits have been suggested to this size, that it was believed that these limits constituted maxima beyond which something essential would be lost in the treatment of the patient. Despite the convictions of those who believed in these limitations it was impossible in a rapidly expanding population such as existed in this country for these limitations to be maintained. The patients had to be cared for. Legislatures were loath to create new institutions and the old ones were added to and grew by these additions from year to year until they far exceeded in size the limitation which was supposed to be an optimum. It might be well, therefore, to look into the question of size to see if there are not some controlling principles that are worth while formulating. In the first place, as I have already indicated, the question of size of the institution and its method of administration can not be separated. The institution of five thousand beds can not be administered in accordance with the same plan of administration as would be employed for a hospital of five hundred beds. That seems to be a basic principle; and one reason, I suspect, that the limitations that I have mentioned were placed upon the growth of mental hospitals was that these hospitals had increased, as I have indicated, by additions, and that the superintendents who originally conducted these institutions of a few hundred beds continued to serve when they became institutions of a thousand or more beds and they did so without changing their methods. They therefore found that their work became increasingly difficult and believed that the increasing difficulty was due, as it was under these circumstances, to the increased size of the institution, and they could see very readily that a little further increase in size would make their work as they were accustomed to do it impossible and would result, therefore, from their point of view, in the neglect of the patients, for the outstanding reason that was given in those days for limiting the number of patients was this: it was held that no institution should be so large that the superintendent could not personally know every patient. Such a principle might easily be expected from the old-time superintendent who conducted his hospital just as he would a big family, and who believed that he ought to be able to answer the questions of all the relatives about each one of his charges, but from the point of view of the development of administration in our great industries such a scheme as this seems to be rather ridiculous. Let us examine it a little more carefully.

In the first place, I have indicated already that medicine was becoming progressively more and more complicated and required a much more complex machinery to make it available for the patient. Specialists of all kinds and technicians and additional physicians had to be added to the staffs of existing institutions in order that the patients could be treated for their various physical ailments. Now to add all the personnel and all the physical equipment that was necessary to bring modern medicine to the patient in the mental hospital was a practical impossibility if this hospital was a hospital of only two or three hundred beds, because it would increase the top cost beyond all reason. No legislature during this period would have thought of appropriating for a state hospital the amount of money that would have been necessary to have maintained any such arrangement. The only way in which it was possible to bring modern medicine to the patient under these circumstances was to increase the size of the institution to such a point that the additional personnel and equipment could be so distributed over a large number of patients that the increase in per capita would be kept at a minimum, and kept at that point which would make it possible to secure appropriations at the per capita rate that was sufficient for the maintenance of this additional equipment. This is the first point that I would make. The second point is that from the point of view of personnel the patient in a great big hospital is infinitely better off than he is in a small hospital. Suppose an institution with two or three hundred beds with only a couple of physicians. These two physicians have to be specialists in every department of medicine or else call in specialists at much added expense to the patient, whereas in large institutions of five thousand or more beds the staff is so large that within its own group it comprises individuals of many different interests, and these various interests are all at the command of any individual sick patient. Further than that, on such a staff the physicians would be appointed because of their special interests. They would be able to maintain them so that they could perform their particular duties for the hospital along the lines of these interests. For instance, there would be the surgeon and the internist as well as the psychiatrist and the psychotherapist.

Aside from the two main points made above which favor institutions of large size, there are other considerations which point in the same direction. For example, in these early days when the hospitals were slowly increasing by the additive process that I have described, there was no adequate personnel in the country for conducting an increased number of institutions; and if the personnel in any particular medical specialty is limited then it is obvious that by a concentration of patients in one place they can receive better care by a limited personnel than they could if they were scattered all over the United States in different institutions. Aside from this, the increased size of the hospital made possible the specialization, as already indicated, of the different members of the staff, which was in harmony with the movement that was going on extra-murally. It meant that a single physician did not have to be able to do everything, that he could be placed at that particular kind of work that best suited his innate capacities and desires, and so a higher degree of efficiency would naturally result from this method of utilizing services. Another feature of the situation is this: that with the constant growth of institutions the standards set for the personnel were constantly being raised so that in the modern large institution there is generally a much greater amount of talent on the medical staff

than in the old institution with its few patients and few physicians,
and the few people throughout the country who are capable of
organizing and maintaining these great medical institutions can be
used to better advantage as heading up large bodies of patients than
if they were scattered about running relatively small plants.   Then in
addition to this, where there is a considerable group of medical men
and they can have their own medical societies competition may be
keen among them and the professional spirit can be maintained at a
higher level and much more easily than it can in isolated institutions
with only two or three physicians.   All of these things have made the
big institution recognized as being on the whole a better place for
the patient, at least the public patient, than the small institution, if
its administrative scheme is properly laid out.   The individual patient
in these large institutions really gets more attention than he would in
a smaller institution rather than less.

I would add here, as I suggested above when I spoke of these
great mental hospitals as wonderful research centers for all kinds
of diseases, particularly for all kinds of physical disease because of
the length of time the patients reside in them, that I think the tendency is beginning to manifest itself, as indicated by the psychopathic
pavilion within the grounds of the general hospital and the psychopathic ward in the general hospital, to do away with the isolation of
the mental patient.   He is being received more and more in general
hospitals and I think the time may come when great medical centers
such as the recent ones that have been built in New York City will
contain regularly their psychopathic departments so that general
medicine and psychiatry will come together in this structural way.
The great state hospital, too, I can see perhaps changing in the same
direction, so that where the supply of land is ample, as it is in some
states, the other public institutions maintained by the state may be
built upon the same property—the tuberculosis hospital, etc., so that
there might be a coming together again of what medical specialism
has separated during the past years, a coming together that might not
only be of scientific importance but of interest socially, adminis-
tratively and economically.

# CHAPTER XVII

## A Modern Hospital for Mental Diseases

From what has already been written the equipment, physical and personal, of the modern hospital for mental diseases might in large part be inferred. I shall, however, undertake very briefly to describe such an institution.

Remembering what has already been said about the state hospital, namely, that through the years it has been the fundamental basis from which modern psychiatry has grown, and recalling the developments of extra-mural psychiatry, I am of the opinion that the state hospital not only continues to be the fundamental source of psychiatric progress but will so continue to be for some years. The improvements, the new discoveries, concepts and theories, will be adopted by the state hospital when they shall have become sufficiently stabilized by experience; and the vast majority of mental patients for a long time to come will necessarily have to be treated in these institutions. What are the functional components of such an institution, based upon the present state of development of psychiatry in its various ramifications?

In the first place, the modern state hospital may be conceived of as an institution which needs to have, in order to obtain the best economic results, somewhere in the neighborhood of five thousand beds. This is necessary, as already intimated, in order that the large number of purely domiciliary patients, patients whose mental disease has become quiescent and who require only to be housed, fed and clothed at minimum expense, can absorb the overhead that is needed to run a modern institution with its various high-powered hospital and laboratory equipment. Such an institution would be made up of the following functional parts: There would be, as already mentioned, a large domiciliary group that would be maintained in a special type of construction that could be administered at the least expense. Then there would be the receiving groups where the proportion of nurses and physicians would necessarily be high and where intensive efforts at therapy would be made. Then there would be the general hospital center for the treatment of somatic disease, which would bear the same relation to the institution as a whole that a municipal hospital bears to a city, so that when anybody in the hospital population becomes sick an ambulance conveys him to the medical and surgical center, which is equipped to deal with somatic disease along the lines of all the medical specialties. Then it is desirable to have, in addition to the medical and surgical center, a hospital for the chronically ill who do not require very expensive hospital care but who do require careful medical supervision in their living, such as the chronic nephritics, the cardiopathics, the diabetics, where these patients may learn to look after their diet and their living, where they can rest large portions of the day in bed and be under medical supervision but not expensive nursing and hospital care. Then in addition there should be a contagious disease pavilion always kept ready for occupancy so that upon the appearance of a contagious disease in the hospital population the patients can be immediately transferred and isolated. In addition to these medical units there should be the necessary building or buildings for caring for the tubercular. Such buildings are necessary not only to give better care for the tubercular but, like the contagious disease building, to prevent infection of the rest of the population. In addition to these units there will naturally be buildings for the convalescent, for the epileptic, and for the more or less disturbed types of patient, especially the more dangerous types, who need a higher percentage of caretakers.

A laboratory should be a part of the equipment of every institution, not only to do the routine examinations of body fluids and tissues which are required in the everyday practice of medicine, but also as a center of research. It should be equipped for all this kind of work and it would be desirable that the personnel should consist of a director who had been especially trained in neuropathology, a bacteriologist who might serve as the public health officer of the hospital reservation as the bacteriologist does at Saint Elizabeths Hospital, and a blood chemist, with the necessary technicians, so that metabolism studies, nutrition studies, ordinary clinical examinations of the body fluids and of the tissues, electro-cardiographic examinations and the like could all be negotiated by the aid of some of the personnel of the laboratory force. The laboratory building might best be next to the general medical and surgical group because of the intimate use of the laboratory by the physicians in this department. The personnel of the medical and surgical department, besides the ordinary equipment of nurses, should include an internist, a resident surgeon, a serologist, and the necessary technicians for

X-ray work and the like; while many of the specialties may be represented by part-time men running a regular outpatient or dispensary department.

The personnel of the medical staff aside from these special departments should be made up, first, of administrative officers of the several services into which the hospital is divided other than those mentioned. These men should be chosen because of their administrative ability. In addition there should be a group of psychotherapists who would be relieved as far as possible from administrative work and would deal primarily with the individual problems of the individual patient. An adequately trained psychologist, who is competent to work out the psychological assets and liabilities of the patient in what I call a " personality profile " and who is fitted by experience to give advice as to occupation, aside from such questions as psychological age, is a very helpful member of the staff. It will be found very practical to refer many problem cases among employees to such a psychologist, as it not infrequently happens even where the civil service is rigidly enforced that defective individuals are certified for employment, or, if not defective, they may have paranoid trends or other psychological conditions that unfit them for the immediate job in which they may be engaged. A social service department, which assists in contacting with patient's homes in order to get information about new patients, and helps the parole patient to adjust to outside conditions and the family to understand him so that his outside adjustment may remain permanent and be followed by discharge, completes the major functional units necessary for a modern institution dealing with mental diseases. It is desirable in addition, of course, that such an institution should not only treat its patients but should be a teaching institution. In the first place, it is desirable that it should have a training school for nurses in which the nurses are trained in the care of mental patients and the personnel of the nursing staff of the hospital provided in this way. It is also highly desirable that such institutions should be teaching centers for nearby medical schools, if there are such, or, if not, that they should give courses for students who are studying sociology, or abnormal psychology, or what not, in nearby universities, and if not this, then that they arrange from time to time programs with medical societies for presenting problems of mental medicine and perhaps arrange speakers for such organizations as parent-teachers associations and others interested in behavior problems. It has long been recognized that the teaching institution furnishes the best treatment for the patient, because an institution which is a center of teaching can not stagnate. It requires that all those who are engaged in lecturing and clinical work shall be kept on their toes with regard to their particular specialty, and the patients necessarily benefit as a result.

Such an institution, with so many functional parts and such a large personnel as indicated above, is, I believe, the best place for a mentally sick individual, because, with a staff of approximately fifty physicians, as such an institution should have, who are devoted to the various aspects of medicine, the patient becomes the beneficiary of the entire group, and in the event of illness free consultation is pretty apt to disclose the real nature of the malady and the proper course to pursue. Inasmuch, however, as there are always conditions that are liable to arise that are unusual in such an institution, surgical conditions, particularly, which require the highly specialized skilled operator in some particular department of surgery, it is desirable that there should be a consulting staff composed of the outstanding physicians in the immediate neighborhood of the hospital. With this set-up, as I have briefly described it, there are very few conditions which can not be adequately met from the medical point of view, all the way from the individual specialty in somatic medicine to the elaborate methods of psychotherapy.

In addition to the highly specialized personnel thus far mentioned the modern hospital requires occupational aides, whose particular function is to distract the introverted, phantasying patient from his day dreams and get him interested in some aspect of reality, so that he may be made accessible, perhaps, for psychotherapeutic talks, or at least for further reality contacts which move in the direction of recovery. There should also be a definite program for initiating the chronic patient, for whom recovery is not expected but who has become a domiciliary problem, into such forms of industry as will be economically and otherwise remunerative to the institution and at the same time keep him healthfully and interestedly occupied. As I have already mentioned, the old state hospital ideal of getting its patients to work on the farm was perhaps one of the best programs that has ever been developed, and it is difficult to improve upon it except in detail and in an institution where the patient is more highly individualized.

Then there should be the bathmasters and the bathmistresses who look after the administration of the various forms of hydrotherapy that may be prescribed—the douches, the packs and the continuous baths, all of which have become so important in the modern hospital and have assisted so largely in doing away with chemical restraint. An institution well equipped with means for the various forms of hydrotherapy is well on the road to practically complete abolishment of the use of sedatives for quieting excited patients.

Then remembering what I have already said, that one of the advantages of the hospital is that the environment is suited to the patient rather than expecting the patient to conform to the environment, there should be developed in each institution a program of recreation and amusement. The amusement consists usually of the time honored weekly dance, which may be interspersed now and again with theatricals, preferably those devised and taken part in by the patients themselves. These entertainments nowadays are supplemented or largely substituted by the moving picture. Musical and theatrical organizations may be formed of employees or patients or both, and may function throughout the year. In the summer time various forms of athletic entertainments and competitions assist in the recreational program that may be advantageously used, field days, baseball games and in particular all games that require mass action, concerted and integrated play by a group of patients.

Then there is the library. Aside from the scientific library, which of course every hospital must have, there should be a circulating library for patients, composed of books of quality and of variety which can be practically the duplicate of the circulating library of the nearby city, as it has been found by experience that the tastes of patients are practically the tastes of the general population. The library adds very much to the contentment of the patient, and if the librarian has initiative she will see that the bed-fast patient gets the opportunity to choose books and magazines by visiting him weekly with an assortment from which he may choose. In the same way those patients who can not go to the amusement hall may be served by means of a portable moving picture apparatus. The amusement hall thus becomes a very important center in these large state hospitals, which, after all, are really municipalities from the point of view of their numerous and complex functions.

Appropriate religious exercises need to be held regularly with clergymen who can respond to the religious needs of the various denominations represented by the patients.

Finally, the whole personnel of the institution should be instructed and trained by regular courses given by the officers of the hospital, and by precept and example, to think of the patient as the central object about which all the machinery of the hospital revolves, and to make it their business to assist individual patients whenever and wherever possible to function in useful and socially acceptable ways either as assistants in some department or activity of the institution or during periods of parole when problems of outside adjustment present themselves. The nurse and the attendant are the nucleus of the therapeutic organization of the institution and their personal relationships with the patient are of the utmost significance; and it is desirable, as far as possible, not only that they should be chosen with the greatest care but that the patients should be selected with reference to the nurses that are to take care of them so that the combination will work with the highest degree of efficiency. The problem here is very different from the problem presented by somatic medicine. Nurses need to have not only tact but a keen intuition that enables them to contact the personality of the patient in an understanding way and to use such contact for the patient's good.

Roughly and briefly speaking, this is the organization of a hospital from the professional, therapeutic and scientific point of view. Nothing has been said about the physical plant, its power house, its steam lines, its electrical equipment, its various industrial departments, the laundry, the commissary department, the carpenter shops, the machine shops, etc., etc.—throughout the whole list of activities which would normally be found in a municipality. All this complicated, interconnected network of machinery makes a fascinatingly interesting environment for the patient, and he should be led to become interested in it as the development of such interest will help him on the road to health. Each of these various activities also represents possibilities for the employment of patients in useful and interesting ways; and the chief engineer and the head plumber and the head electrician, the head carpenter, and all the rest of them, should understand that their outstanding duty is to assist patients who may be assigned to them to make industrial and social adjustments. In this way the hospital becomes in every smallest portion of it an adjunct in the treatment of the patient and needs to be used in that way. The state hospital, therefore, as a whole, with its extensive grounds and farms, its many departments of activity, its thousands of patients and its hundreds of employees, becomes a special type of social unit constructed and maintained in its various activities with the specific objective of assisting the individual mentally ill patient back to health. Viewed in this way it will be seen that it constitutes a unique bit of machinery designed for therapeutic purposes and that as such it utilizes all of the possibilities and potentialities of a complex social unit, for example, from the small needle and thread which may be used to sew up a scalp wound to the highly complex social organization which ultimately may pass upon the acceptability or otherwise of an individual's conduct.

This whole organization, which must be considered to be a rather gigantic affair for the purposes for which it exists, is all directed by the superintendent for the one end of the welfare of the patient. Probably almost anyone who would read this account would be inclined to think that the patients were dealt with *en masse,* that they were brought into the institution by the hundreds, classified into this or that group and dealt with as groups, and to a very large extent this was so with the old state hospital. But as psychiatry has advanced during the past generation it has become increasingly evident that whatever might be accomplished by this group method it was, theoretically at least, highly important to get at the problem of the individual, and the organization of these institutions now is directed to the purpose of individual therapy. For example, such devices as cafeterias are being introduced, not only because they make the patients better satisfied with the food but where they are properly conducted they give the patient a certain amount of individual choice. They make him feel that he is not just one of a large number, but that he continues to maintain his independence. In the same way patients are permitted to choose the material of which their clothing is to be made, and to say something about how it shall be fabricated. The beauty parlor is a recent development along this line of helping to maintain the individuality of the patient. The so-called " back wards," or the wards to which the more or less violent, destructive and untidy patients tend to gravitate, have received special treatment, on the theory that if such wards can be prevented from developing just so much would be accomplished toward preventing the extreme symptoms of mental disease which are found in these localities. Mental disease as it occurs in the state hospital is a regressive phenomenon, and these back wards are invitations to those who have regressive tendencies to develop in their direction. They beckon the patient, in other words, to an environment where no restraint is required, where all the fences are down and self-control such as is required by the standards of society needs no longer to be exercised. The old institutions neglected these wards and they developed in accordance with the general tendency of the patient's illness. Now the effort is to prevent regression to such low levels. And so in all these ways and in many others the individual patient, even in an institution where there are thousands of patients, receives individual attention. In the old state hospital the individual attention came from the attendants and the supervisors. Now it comes from the medical staff and results in some sort of therapy being addressed to each patient's needs.

# CHAPTER XVIII

## The Future

I suppose it is the lot of every superintendent of an institution for mental disease to be asked a certain number of times each year whether in his opinion "insanity" is on the increase. Such a query is impossible to answer, primarily because it is impossible to ask. The very question itself involves concepts which, in the form in which the question is put, have no real meaning. "Insanity," as I have often explained, is purely a social and legal term and means a degree of maladjustment which is sufficient to cause society, through the operation of the machinery set up for that purpose, to segregate the individual. It is a term, therefore, obviously relative to the social conditions and the social standards of conduct which may happen to prevail at any particular time or any particular place. Mental disease may progress very far in an individual who lives on an isolated farm in a very thinly populated district, whereas mental disease of much less pronounced character may cause the individual's apprehension and detention if it occurs in an individual living in the thickly populated area of a metropolitan district. "Insanity" used in this way, therefore, must have a constantly changing meaning as society becomes progressively more and more complicated and population more and more congested. Then, again, we have had statistics of mental disease in this country only since 1880 and this covers altogether too brief a period to be of much value in determining what the trend may be; and yet during this period not only has the actual number of mentally ill patients confined in public institutions increased very greatly but it has increased much more rapidly than the population, so that there is ample reason for being apprehensive as to the future. At the present time there are approximately 400,000 mentally ill patients confined in the various institutions throughout the United States, and the statisticians are telling us that in 1970, only 38 years hence, when the United States will have a stable population of 150,000,000, there will then be 950,000 mentally ill patients in hospitals. In other words, with an increase in population of approximately 20 per cent there will be, in round numbers, 100 per cent increase in the number of mentally ill patients in hospitals. This is indeed an alarming state of affairs to look forward to. When translated into dollars and cents it means an enormous burden for the state to carry; and when we consider that in all probability the number of feebleminded and epileptics and other types of inadequate personalities is probably at least as many again, the burden becomes rather appalling. What is the answer to such a situation? Are we simply to go on building hospitals and taking care of those who can not carry on outside, those who can not stand on their own feet? It is probably the most important public health problem that confronts us today.

In order to understand this situation it is necessary to analyze to some extent the meaning of these figures. In the first place, in all probability, it does not necessarily mean, as some people seem to be inclined to believe, that the race is degenerating rapidly and that ultimately the burden of the dependents will be so great as to break down the whole structure of civilization. In the brief space of the forty years covered by my personal experience I have seen the state hospital emerge from being an institution against which all sorts of criticisms were directed and around which all sorts of suspicions revolved, an institution in other words which was far from having the confidence of the public, and become a hospital for the care of certain kinds of sick individuals which was sought by the patient and by the patient's relatives as a natural source of relief from their difficulties. From being an isolated community engaged in the somewhat questionable practice of taking care of the so-called " insane," being suspected of all sorts of ulterior motives and of being subject to improper influences by retaining individuals who were not " insane " at the behest of wealthy and influential individuals who desired their sequestration, it has gained the confidence of the people it serves, not only by doing a progressively better and better job for the patients it received, as the years went by, but also by extending its helping hand beyond its walls through its social service department and by means of establishing mental hygiene clinics in the various towns throughout the district it served and so attempting to help those patients who were on parole or had been discharged and felt that they were again slipping, or entirely new cases who sought the clinic for advice and guidance. In this way the state hospital is gradually becoming a tower of strength in the community it serves, and because of the dropping away of the suspicions which the community used to have regarding it and the substitution of confidence patients seek its help in much greater numbers and this is undoubtedly one of the reasons for the apparent increase in the number of mental cases throughout the country. The history of the mental hospital in this respect is not essentially different from the history of the general hospital. I was born and brought up within half a block of such an institution and I well remember in my boyhood days the stories that were told about the way in which patients were treated in that institution. It was generally believed by many of the ignorant who lived in the neighborhood that when a patient in the opinion of the doctors could not get well he was given " the black bottle," in other words, that he was quietly put out of the way. Just as the general hospital has survived these beliefs and has grown into a benefaction, so now the hospital for mental disease can look back upon a similar history and realize that it is only now emerging from the operation of just such impediments to its higher social usefulness.

When all this is said, however, it does not lead us very far in the direction of solving the problem as stated in the opening paragraphs of this chapter. We have all the more reason because of these facts for believing that the load of mental illness will increase rather than decrease, because people will be conscious of what constitutes mental illness in themselves as well as in others and will seek in increasing numbers for relief from the handicaps of this sort of sickness. What are the prospects that the future holds forth for being able to meet these conditions by any reasonable expenditure of energy and money? Is it going to be possible, or must we look forward to ever increasing burdens which will finally become intolerable?

Many scientifically minded individuals have been alarmed by this condition, and many books have been written and many suggestions made and many remedies outlined. One of the things which the superintendent of a hospital for mental illness hears almost as frequently as he hears the question as to whether he believes " insanity " is on the increase is the question as to whether he does not believe it would be better to put all these unfortunate people quietly and pain-lessly out of the way. Euthanasia, in other words, is the suggested remedy for this tremendous social burden. I do not know how others answer this question, but I always say that of course, in the first place, such a suggestion can not be considered simply because in this day and age it would be impossible, but that even if it were possible I personally should not want to live in a society that dealt with its unfortunates in such a way. Such methods of treatment would unloose the sadistic tendencies which we already have sufficient difficulty in keeping repressed and which with all the armamentarium of the present civilization we do not succeed in repressing all of the time by any means and which when they do get loose create such terrific havoc as we have recenty passed through in the World War. With " insanity " having no specific meaning and being incapable of being defined, it can easily be imagined how a civilization, if that word can be used, which had gone on the loose as regards sadistic tendencies could easily find ways to determine that anyone who opposed it was " insane " and apply euthanasia to him. As soon as one begins to think through any such proposition its utter inpracticability, to say nothing of its danger, immediately presents itself.

A somewhat similar suggestion is that of the eugenists, who outline a program of sterilization by which they would prevent the birth of individuals doomed to become socially dependent as a result of mental defect or disease. We have had in this country for some years sterilization laws in many states, but for the most part they are inoperative, at least they are inoperative so far as having any effect upon this great problem is concerned. They embody, as I see it, very little else than a wish to improve the conditions of society, but good intentions can not take the place of actual knowledge which we do not possess in this instance. The sterilization laws in most of the states are practically inoperative and where they are enforced they are enforced by individuals who are in no position to know anything of the scientific aspects of the problem; and when one looks into these scientific aspects one is confronted by the fact that after all nobody knows enough to predict what the progeny of a given individual's germ plasm may be like. It is rather extraordinary that all of these sterilization laws have reference to the individual, the idea being evidently to destroy or to terminate a bad strain of germ plasm, whereas, so far as I know, no effort at prediction of what sort of progeny can be expected can be made with reference to the make-up of any single individual. One has to take into consideration also the make-up of that individual's mate. But be that as it may, there is no existing information, so far as I know, that warrants sterilization as a solution for this problem. It is barely possible that some effect might be made upon the number of incompetents if it were carried out on the stupendous scale that has been suggested and which involves the immediate sterilization of some ten millions of the present population. But this, on its face, is an absurd suggestion. I am not sure but that sterilization may persist and have some functions that are worth while, but its uses will necessarily be very much restricted and will have no effect upon this great problem unless our knowledge is very greatly increased over what it is at present. The simplistic ideals upon which the theory of sterilization is founded must give place to actual scientific knowledge, and this as yet has not occurred.

While discussing this point of attempting to solve the problem of the future by a process of destroying the possibilities of creating diseased individuals in the next generation, I may mention a fact which is generally overlooked, and that is that the differential death rate runs against these defective and psychotic individuals. The United States Census reports show that the defective and psychotic individuals in the public institutions throughout the country have a death rate from six to seven times as great as individuals of the same age outside. So it would seem that whether we develop a program of sterilization or not, Nature does have effective means at her disposal for correcting serious dysgenic situations as they arise.

Then one must remember with regard to the defective or the feebleminded that, to some extent at least, these terms also must be considered as relative, that even if it were possible to destroy all germ plasm which today is regarded as defective and create a superior race in accordance with the ideals of the eugenicists, still the probabilities are that there would be about as much distance between those at the top and those at the bottom in such a race as there is today. Be that as it may, one can not help but think of the future in terms of the past so far as the conquering of disease is concerned. The contagious and infectious diseases are conquered or conquerable. We either have largely eliminated them or else we know how to do it and it only remains to devise means that are socially workable. Syphilis, for example, is very easily prevented on paper but practically it becomes a problem of stupendous difficulties. Nevertheless, life has been very greatly prolonged in recent years, but the sorts of diseases that we are discussing, the mental diseases, have not been lessened. Tuberculosis is apparently on the decline but mental disease because life has been prolonged seems to be statistically on the increase, for people are living into the period in which certain types of mental disease develop. We can not help, however, hoping that some day we may know enough about all of the problems that are involved so that we can have a civilization the individual units of which have a reasonable expectancy of a long life free from serious illness, with the prospect of death coming gently at the expiration of many years of usefulness. But when such an objective may be attained no one, I presume, would be hazardous enough to guess. As the matter stands today, the future of the race from this point of view is in the lap of the gods.

There are certain immediate objectives that it is possible to take hold of at the present time, however, that may be mentioned. In the first place, it is quite obvious that if our concept of mental disease is correct it is of great importance that the patient should seek competent assistance at the earliest possible date. This is happening more and more as the hospitals are becoming institutions to be sought rather than avoided. With the new concepts of these diseases that have developed and are developing it is possible that therapeutic efforts in the future will be more effective and efficient than they have been in the past. Furthermore, it is possible that the wide popularization of psychology and psychiatry which has been taking place now from the beginning of this century may ultimately make it possible for people of quite limited means to live more safely and happily outside an institution. This is what I have in mind: Mental defectives, as I often say, are much more nearly 100 per cent efficient than the rest of us. A deficient boy may be taught to do a certain task that is well within his powers and do it in a certain way and do it every day and do it with equal thoroughness upon each occasion. He varies little from day to day. His accomplishments are machine-like in their predictability and accuracy. In this machine age individuals that can be taught to do definite things with this automatic certainty of results, and who, I may add parenthetically, are contented and happy in such tasks with only an occasional word of praise and encouragement, ought to find a place of usefulness if they were understood. The unfortunate part, however, is that they are not understood. Mary, a defective girl, may be taught accurately to set the table three times a day for a family of four people, and she will do this task perfectly upon each occasion. But let a stranger be invited to dinner and the fifth place be required, and the whole structure comes falling down like a house of cards. She is perfectly dazed and confused at this new adjustment required of her. She can not make the grade. Now if the mistress understands Mary this is merely a passing incident but if, as is probably and unfortunately more often true, the mistress loses her temper and gets mad at Mary then matters are made worse, perhaps hopelessly worse. Mary loses her job, she gets no recommendation, and thrown upon her own she is perfectly helpless in an unsympathetic, non-understanding world. I have long thought that some day it might be possible that these defective types might be appreciated at their real values and find a place under the sun, and that society instead of acting like Mary's mistress would undertake to see that they received some sort of protection. This can be done outside an institution, as is already being demonstrated by institutions for the feebleminded in this country; but progress is slow and in the meantime if we have to keep taking these people into institutions this sort of thing certainly can be effected there. The main things that stand in the way of doing this is the extent of original capital investment and the interference with local labor conditions which might result.

As thus far sketched the future does not seem to offer any very glowing possibilities, or at least the near future. Treatment results have probably not greatly increased the number of recoveries except in so far as more acute situations are received, and are received earlier, while the prospects of a scientifically justifiable eugenics program are too remote to expect relief from that quarter for a long time. But there are certain aspects of the problem which ordinarily escape notice and to which it is worth while to call attention. In the first place, during the period that an individual is confined in an institution for mental disease he is as effectively sterilized as if he had been operated upon. In this way, therefore, the increasing number of patients who are institutionalized has much the same effect as a sterilizing program; and when compared with the number that are actually being sterilized at present it is much more effective, because only very, very few patients are now being operated upon. The institution, therefore, acts as a means of accelerating natural selection; and the more defectives and the more sick people that are removed from the community, the more nearly is the community a society of reasonably efficient and reasonably healthy people.

It is hardly fair to leave the question of treatment with only the few words above. It must be appreciated that an enormous amount of new information has been accumulated during the present century, and, what is still more important, the door has been opened for infinitely more. The psychoanalysts are only beginning to tackle the problem of the major psychoses, and while no predictions are warranted at the present time still it must be obvious that increasing information with regard to this group of diseases will lead to more intelligent care and treatment; and while it may not be possible, and probably will not be, to undertake the psychotherapy of every patient admitted to a mental institution, still general principles of treatment will undoubtedly be worked out in the future which will be more effective than those now being used.

This question of the treatment of the psychoses should not be left without a word regarding paresis. Paresis, of course, is the late result of an infection, but practically 10 per cent of the patients in our public institutions for mental disease are paretics. Until recently we had considered this disease absolutely hopeless, every patient dying after a course of varying length; but with the advent of the treatment of this disease by malaria this whole picture has been radically changed, and it is not uncommon now for patients to go back into the community as efficient and self-supporting citizens.*

Perhaps when psychiatric principles have been more fully developed as controlling factors in dealing with the so-called criminal population similar results will take place here. A large proportion of the inmates of various penal institutions are either mentally defective or disordered in some way, and, as experience has shown through the years, the turning of these people back into the community is just inviting a repetition of the events which led to their original incarceration. Just as the growth of state hospitals in some parts of the country has been coincident with the gradual diminution in the population of the poor houses, so it is conceivable that the state hospital should either take over the population that otherwise would go into the prisons, or that the psychiatrist in taking over the prisons should turn them into institutions which are more nearly like the state hospitals and should in the same way deal with the inmates from the point of view of their social adaptability and not from the point of view of an arbitrarily determined sentence.

There is one change which the future may see effected which is dependent largely upon economic pressure, namely, the more effective employment of patients in these large institutions. As the matter stands today every effort is made to employ the maximum number of patients on the theory that employment is therepeutically worth while, but it is essential that the products of this employment be all consumed by the institution. There is a great deal of simple work to be done, such as polishing floors and washing windows, which can be done by the more defective or deteriorated patients; there is a great deal of laboring work to be done, such as the digging of tunnels and the shoveling of coal, which can be done by the more powerfully muscled patients; and there is a great deal of more intelligent work

* This treatment was first introduced into this country at Saint Elizabeths Hospital, where the first patient was inoculated with malaria in December of 1922. See Medical Research Bulletin No. 8, Saint Elizabeths Hospital, U. S. Department of the Interior. U. S. Government Printing Office, Washington, 1932.

that can be done either in the various machine shops in connection with the several industries or in the business offices of the hospital. There is also a considerable amount of work in actual manufacturing which can be done, as, for instance, in the making of shoes and brushes and clothing.  But all of this, as I have already said, has to be used by the institution.  The outside markets can not be utilized for disposing of these things.  Labor conditions are such as to make this impossible.  Now in the hospitals throughout the United States hundreds of thousands of dollars, millions of dollars in fact, of products are fabricated every year by the patient population.  During the last fiscal year the value of the products fabricated in Saint Elizabeths Hospital, calculated at market values, was in round numbers $800,000, and yet in my opinion the actual value of patients' labor has nowhere reached its limits.  We could produce here easily twice, probably three times as much, maybe more, if we could install in the hospital modern methods of mass production and had a market for our goods.  At present, for the most part, hospitals use only primitive methods of manufacture in order to keep their patients employed.  Modern machinery would change all this very rapidly. Whether the time will ever come when this will be possible I do not know but I suspect that the increasing number of patients who have to be cared for and the increasing cost of their care will ultimately produce an economic pressure that will tend to move in this direction. People will begin to see that the only salvation, economically at least, is to have these institutions produce sufficiently to assist materially in the cost of their upkeep.  It is possible that in the future all public institutions will be gathered into great medical centers.  For example, if the state tuberculosis hospital were on the same grounds as the state hospital for mental disease, then the milk and the eggs and the vegetables which are raised by the patients at the state hospital over and beyond what they consume themselves could go to the tuberculosis hospital.  And so here would be created a market which does not exist now in the several states.  After this was done, however, there might still be a surplus which could be sold in the open market; and I have a suspicion that with the continuing of restricted immigration the labor organizations might be sympathetic towards such a program, as they are already beginning to be sympathetic towards the program of employing prisoners.  This is at least a practical suggestion along lines which may easily be effected. The future, perhaps the near future, will show.  In addition to this scheme and as a further elaboration, it would be perfectly possible in a state that has a number of state hospitals, such as New York or Massachusetts, to distribute its skilled workers among its different institutions to the best economic and industrial advantage, so that they could concentrate upon special products.

Psychiatry, as already indicated, has reached out in many directions and has become important in connection with the solution of many significant problems. As I see the field of psychiatry extending in this way I am reminded of the principles that underlie the administration of the gradually enlarging institution. Just as at first the growing institution centralizes all of its authority in one office, so the growth of psychiatry is being centralized in the psychiatrist; but just as the institutional community gets too large to have its administration all take place from one central point and there has to come about a certain amount of decentralization, so the same thing will happen in the field of psychiatry and the principles will have to be put in operation by people who are not primarily psychiatrists. I have this in mind in advocating more extensive instruction in this branch of medicine in medical colleges. I feel that every physician ought to go into the community as well grounded in psychiatry as he is in the principles of obstetrics, pediatrics, surgery, and other medical specialties. In this way he will be able to deal with perhaps the majority of psychiatric problems with which he is faced in his practice, requiring to call in a specialist only in exceptional cases. This is the way he practices medicine with reference to the other medical specialties, and there is no reason why it should not be his method with regard to psychiatry. And so in this sense every physician would have a psychiatric foundation; and whether he goes into the school, or the college, or the police department, or the prison, or the factory, or wherever he goes, he will carry this information and apply it in his daily work. This is comparable to the decentralization process referred to in administration, while the great centers of psychiatric activity like the state hospitals will continue to furnish new facts as a result of research these facts will be applied more and more widely by an ever increasing number of individuals.

# CHAPTER XIX

## CONCLUSION

We have finally come to the end of our narrative and it remains only to sum up a few of the more important points and to add a few words in conclusion.

I have not undertaken in this work to trace the history of the "insane." I have only attempted to tell something of what has happened during the past forty years. But even in this relatively short span of time practically everything that is of outstanding importance and significance has in reality occurred. While the humanitarian era is arbitrarily thought of as having been ushered in by Pinel in the last of the eighteenth century, still forty years ago there were conditions in some of the public institutions of the United States that were quite as atrocious as those which Pinel undertook to correct in Paris. Over the length and breadth of the country the "insane" were found in considerable numbers in jails and prisons and alms-houses, and in conditions of hopeless neglect in their own homes. Poorhouse keepers were priding themselves on the cheapness with which they could feed these unfortunate persons. Asylums were confining them in camisoles and locking them up in strong-rooms, and sometimes in cages very much like wild animals, while it was not entirely unheard of to have them housed in filthy, decrepit shacks without light, ventilation or adequate sanitation, and sometimes actually in chains. What I have tried to do in the pages of this book is to tract not chronologically but functionally the changes that have occurred from this medieval rest in our social organization to the advanced positions of the scientific salient of the present day. It is of course unfortunately true that many primitive conditions still exist, and it is also true that no one who is forward-thinking is satisfied with what has been accomplished. In other words, there are still evils to correct and progress is still taking place. But from the hideous conditions of medievalism to which I have just referred to the best conditions found in our modern hospitals is a gigantic stride and involves radical changes of thought and feeling and attitude, and improvement in methods, together with the utilization of

[148]

the facts which have been disclosed as a result of the advance of science.

It is true that as we examine the conditions about us and attempt to change them for the better we gain the feeling that man progresses with exceeding slowness, that tremendous efforts extending over long periods produce only minute results. On the other hand, as we look back upon what has been accomplished we are invariably surprised at how far we have come along the path of progress. I suspect that these opposite feelings are dependent upon the fact that while we do personally exert ourselves tremendously, very little of the progress that takes place is really due to these personal exertions of ours. Somehow or other things come to pass, and it is always questionable just how much we have to do with the final results. Do we effect them, or, on the other hand, are those of us who are most fortunate capable of feeling ourselves into the trends of the times and moving along with them, largely passive agents in this progressive change? However that may be, no one can doubt that this tremendous change that I have described has taken place; but I might add that probably very few really appreciate its outstanding significance. The things which have been happening in the past forty years and which I have described in the pages of this book, are the beginning stages of what may be perhaps the most significant thing that has ever happened to man in the course of his life on earth. They are the beginnings of man's understanding of man, his first efforts to come to grips with himself, to face the realities of his instinctual drives as they lie buried beneath the disguises that modern civilization demands. This function of the mind which has now only for the first time been stirred to conscious activity I have expressed elsewhere as follows :*

" No adequate understanding of the present status of the study of the human mind can be reached, as indeed might be said of any other scientific subject, without some knowledge of the historical aspects of the subject. And I may remind you in this connection that it is only very recently that the study of the human mind in its various reaches has escaped from the limitations of its associations with philosophy, theology and morals and has finally become, in my opinion, a biological science which undertakes to investigate and explain not only the outwardly observable behavior of living beings but the circumstances in that world

* The Study of the Mind. Science, Vol. 76, No. 1961, July 29, 1932, pp. 90–92.

within us, which can only be approached by methods of introspection, which are of such apparent significance in connection with our behavior as to make it seem dependent on our ways of thinking and feeling.

" It has been known for many years that the perception of the outer world was more or less modified by the individual, differently in different cases; and the personal equation which was developed as a corrective device for doing away with or at least minimizing the distortion that was inevitable, and which was shown in the different results obtained by different observers in recording the same phenomena, stands as a concrete expression of the realization of this fact. But such variations as one finds in this field of scientific observation, variations which showed up in the reading of scientific instruments, while it is important, is, to put it mildly, of minor significance as compared with the distortions of the universe about us which from our point of view we read into the perceptions of primitive man, of the child, and of the mentally diseased, and which as mass phenomena have invaded civilization from time to time in such expressions, for example, as the belief in witchcraft which swept over Europe, persisted for some hundreds of years, and cost hundreds of thousands if not millions of lives. All these groups of phenomena are manifestations of the distortion of reality as it filters through the individual and is interpreted by him upon the basis of his background of experience, both individually and racially.

" The researches within the present century in the field of psychopathology have had as one distinct objective, among others, the correction of these distortions with a realization, quite naturally, of the philosophical implication that after all the universe is for us as we perceive it but with no longer the necessity for being controlled, inhibited and prevented from progress by such a hypothesis; for if this statement of philosophy is accepted at its face value it would mean that progress in the interpretation of the facts of reality was either impossible, or, if not that, at least outside of our control, that nothing we could do would affect the net results one way or the other. Progress voluntarily aspired to by means or methods intelligently addressed to that end would be nothing more nor less than an attempt to accomplish the impossible, but the remarkable fact is that man is able to accomplish the impossible or at least what seems to be the impossible. I might perhaps better say that life in its evolutionary and developmental progress stands out as an example of the accomplishment of the impossible, and man may continue to progress if he has the courage to discard limiting theories and go bravely forward, even though what he seeks may seem to him at the time unattainable.

" The mind of man has in the present century come into its

own for the first time as a worthy subject of scientific study and investigation; and if some of the investigations and some of the studies made appear to lead to rather unacceptable results, or results which do not seem to measure up to the requirements of the standards which have been attained in other scientific disciplines, it is, in my opinion, only because we are dealing with an infinitely complex group of problems and we are only beginning to attempt to deal with them in a scientific manner, free from prejudice, superstition and the like; and the important thing is not so much the accomplishment in a specific instance as the fact that sincere efforts are being made by an ever-increasing body of enthusiastic students. Even though I indicate the situation in these rather discouraging words, still enough has been accomplished to act as a sufficient stimulus for the high adventure of further discoveries, because of the tremendous importance and significance of this field as already disclosed. For example, we are beginning to feel very definitely—some of us at least—that the phenomena at what I call the psychological level of functioning of the living being, while to be sure they are intangible, imponderable and invisible, are nevertheless somehow to be related in our thinking to the manifestations of energy with which we are more familiar in the physical world. The psyche is being considered as an organ the function of which, expressed in its most generic form, is the equalizing of stresses and the releasing of tensions, with the necessary tendency to bring to pass a state of equilibrium—not a static equilibrium but a dynamic equilibrium. And as we undertake to evaluate various states of mind we can not escape from the necessity of measuring them over against the stimuli which have released them and forming some sort of judgment as to the quantitative relations between the two. We see, for example, such quantitative relations, although to be sure we have no means of measuring them with accuracy, between the depth of grief of an individual over the loss by death of a beloved friend or relative and the importance and significance of that friend or relative in the life of the survivor. We see very definite quantitative relations between the feeling of guilt and the nature of the act which has excited it; and when we realize in such instances as this latter, for example, that such a reaction is based upon an inner standard against which the individual measures his conduct, and that that inner standard is received from the cultural environment in which the individual was raised and becomes such a standard by being built into the psyche, you will perhaps understand what I mean when I say that I believe in the last analysis that the psyche may be considered as an environmental inclusion in a sense not dissimilar from that in which the blood is considered to have been originally the environmental inclusion of a droplet of sea-water, which subsequently became the circulating medium for the transportation of various substances from one part of the body to another.

" If such an hypothesis, or perhaps it might better be called a speculation, should ultimately prove out, it would then mean what again we already have definite hints of: that the laws which govern in the physical world and with which we are to a certain extent familiar would be determined to govern in this apparently more tenuous and immaterial world, the world within. We would find that the relation between stimuli and mental states, as already indicated, was a quantitative one; for example, the relation between a frustration and a compensation. We would see analogies with scientific laws with which we are already familiar, and to which we would become progressively less able to remain blind.

" If all the above things represent a fair statement of how we may consider mental events in their relation to other events in the cosmos, then it can be further understood how significant this particular class of events has become for an adequate understanding of the most important aspects in which we relate ourselves to our environment, namely, those inter-personal relations which have to do with our contacts with other human beings and upon the nature of which it may easily be said depends the whole future course of civilization. Civilization is a matter of the psychology of the peoples functioning at a social level of integration, and no adequate understanding of the forces that are involved can be had unless this fact is appreciated, and we can not expect to guide these forces into constructive channels unless we have this information.

" While it is true that this program contemplates a procedure which looks a little as if man had the problem on his hands of raising himself by his own boot-straps, nevertheless, as I have said, this impossible performance is just precisely what he has proved himself in the past capable of doing. And so it would seem that the reception of psychology into the realm of the biological sciences, the appreciation of man from this point of view functioning as a social unit, and the attempt to fathom the intricacies of the human psyche by the development of methods of research in this field, are worthy, significant and important developments in the world of science which need to be aided, abetted and encouraged by all those who in their own particular fields may have reached a higher degree of perfection both in the observation, description and interpretation of their facts, and in the development of ways and means for their uncovering."

From the above it is easy to see the significance of what I often emphasize—that progress up to the beginning of this century has been progress in the development of man's environment. Science has complicated this beyond the possibilities of belief of a century ago, but during all this time it would seem that man has paid correspondingly less attention to himself and finally he discovers himself among all these enormous powers which he has at his disposal and which science has made possible and is very properly alarmed at the possibilities to which his newly found powers may be turned, for, like everything else, they are ambivalent and as powerful for evil as they are for good. An electric current may be switched into a city and light the streets and the homes and be a beneficent force, or it may be switched into the electric chair and destroy life.

When he thinks of these possibilities which the mind has of distorting the environment, the psychiatrist, at least, has learned to distrust the opinions and the statements of others. He finds it impossible to take others at their face value, and he therefore necessarily has to try to read between the lines in order to extract the true meaning. By that same token, too, he has learned to distrust even himself, so that he has to think twice and be sure, not that he is not fooling someone else but that he is not fooling himself. These are not new developments in the history of man but they are new developments to have been dealt with scientifically. They were before the property of everybody, more or less, particularly perhaps the diplomat; but now everybody must face these possible distorting influences as we meet them in ourselves and others, and one can look forward to the possibilities that a larger recognition of these facts will bring to pass. It will be less and less easy for political demagogues, for example, to fool the people by their perfervid orations. We see here, too, the reasonableness of the psychoanalytic point of view that requires of each individual who is to become an analyst that he himself be first analyzed, have his own blind spots eliminated before he undertakes to deal with others. Every psychiatrist has had the experience of seeing lives wrecked by the vicious influences of other people, influences which perhaps were exercised with the best of intentions but which nevertheless were distorting in their effects. So that a larger, profounder knowledge by man of himself will perhaps have a tendency to check these distorting influences and reduce them to a minimum, for obviously they can never be entirely done away with.

Psychiatry, then, to my mind, presents in its development the results attained by man in his efforts to understand himself and as such it bids fair for some time to come to present in its results some

of the most important and significant additions to scientific knowledge.   It was the first medical specialty that perforce had to deal
with man as a whole and not with some particular organ, and it was
the first to appreciate to the full the practical significance of man's
distortion not only of the environment but of himself in his thinking
and feeling processes.   It therefore strikes at the very heart of the
most important and significant problem that is presented to man,
namely, the problem of himself, and so its development in the future
will be of the utmost significance.

# NERVOUS AND MENTAL DISEASE MONOGRAPH SERIES

Edited by DRS. SMITH ELY JELLIFFE and WILLIAM A. WHITE

## Numbers Issued